MEDICAL DEVICES AND EQUIPMENT

MEDICAL IMAGING

PROCEDURES, TECHNIQUES AND APPLICATIONS

MEDICAL DEVICES AND EQUIPMENT

Additional books in this series can be found on Nova's website under the Series tab.

Additional e-books in this series can be found on Nova's website under the e-books tab.

BIOMEDICAL DEVICES AND THEIR APPLICATIONS

Additional books in this series can be found on Nova's website under the Series tab.

Additional e-books in this series can be found on Nova's website under the e-books tab.

MEDICAL DEVICES AND EQUIPMENT

MEDICAL IMAGING

PROCEDURES, TECHNIQUES AND APPLICATIONS

MAURIZIO D'ELIA
AND
AMEDEO MADAFFARI
EDITORS

Nova Science Publishers, Inc.
New York

For permission to use material from this book please contact us:
Telephone 631-231-7269; Fax 631-231-8175
Web Site: http://www.novapublishers.com

Additional color graphics may be available in the e-book version of this book.

LIBRARY OF CONGRESS CATALOGING-IN-PUBLICATION DATA

ISBN: 978-1-62081-049-1
Library of Congress Control Number: 2012931074

Published by Nova Science Publishers, Inc. † New York

CONTENTS

PREFACE

In this book, the authors discuss the procedures, techniques and applications of medical imaging; which creates images of the human body for clinical purposes or medical science. Topics discussed in this compilation include the use of whole-body fluorine-18-fluorodeoxyglucose positron emission tomography in patients with large-vessel vasculitis and sarcoidosis; medical image registration; radiological techniques in medical imaging; electrical impedance tomography (EIT); imaging of brain function with PET and its role in aphasia research; and real-time functional magnetic resonance imaging.

Chapter 1 - Objective: To review the emerging role of positron emission tomography (PET) and positron emission tomography/computed tomography (PET/CT) with Fluorine-18-fluorodeoxyglucose (FDG) in patients with large-vessel vasculitis (LVV). Methods: A literature search of published studies regarding whole-body FDG-PET and PET/CT in patients with LVV was performed. Results: Main findings of the scientific literature are reported and discussed. Conclusions: FDG-PET and PET/CT are useful imaging methods in the initial diagnosis, in the assessment of activity and extent of disease in patients with LVV. The correlation between FDG-PET findings and serological levels of inflammatory markers as well as the usefulness of FDG-PET and PET/CT in evaluating treatment response remain unclear; it appears that there is a superiority of FDG-PET and PET/CT over conventional imaging methods in the diagnosis of LVV, but not in assessing disease activity under immunosuppressive treatment, in predicting relapse or in evaluating vascular complications.

Chapter 2 - Image registration that is used to reconstruct 3D structure of tissues from a series of images is an important topic in medical image analysis.

However, it becomes a difficult challenge for image registration due to a variety of inherent factors, such as color difference and geometry discrepancy. In this chapter, a robust registration algorithm is proposed to automatically reconstruct 3D volume data from histological images. It mainly contains three procedures, including wavelet-based feature extraction, analytic robust point matching (ARPM), and registration refinement by modified Levenberg-Marquardt algorithm (FMLM). The concept that features could exist in multiscale is used to extract true feature points. The ARPM registration algorithm is then proposed to speedily accomplish the registration of two point sets with different size by simultaneously evaluating the spatial correspondence and geometrical transformation. Finally, a FMLM method is used to further refine registration results and achieve subpixel accuracy. The performance of proposed method is evaluated in comparison with several well-known approaches. The results indicate that the proposed method is a robust and fast method in image registration.

Chapter 3 - Objective: to review the emerging role of whole-body positron emission tomography (PET) and positron emission tomography / computed tomography (PET/CT) with Fluorine-18-Fluorodeoxyglucose (FDG) in patients with sarcoidosis. Methods: A literature search of published studies regarding whole-body FDG-PET and PET/CT in patients with sarcoidosis was performed. Results: Main findings of the scientific literature are reported and discussed. Conclusions: Positive FDG-PET findings should be interpreted with caution in differentiating sarcoidosis from other inflammatory diseases and malignant abnormalities. FDG-PET seems to be a very useful molecular imaging method in assessing disease activity, in staging and identifying occult sites, and in monitoring treatment response in patients with sarcoidosis. FDG-PET shows a better diagnostic accuracy compared to Gallium-67 scintigraphy in patients with sarcoidosis, in addition to several practical advantages.

Chapter 4 – There are several methods largely implemented and employed for daily medical imaging aimed to non-invasive early prevention and/or disease diagnosis. This chapter is dedicated to radiological techniques in medical imaging. It concerns the interaction of ionizing radiation with patient. From a general point of view, it may be possible to characterise radiological medical imaging techniques in two different categories, the first one devoted to structural information to get anatomical images, whereas there are other types of methods dedicated to obtain functional information in order to provide some metabolic patient characterization. It has been previously presented by several authors that this kind of imaging techniques maybe suitably modeled and eventually improved by means of both theoretical and experimental approaches. This chapter will concentrate on analytical along with corresponding numerical models, both integrated in dedicated algorithms capable of handling main physical phenomena related with radiation transport and interaction processes. Detailed descriptionwill be presented about the main features regarding radiation transport modeling for radiological purposes. As example, the developed medical imaging approaches will be implemented and preliminary tested for conventional absorption contrast anatomical imaging, like radiography, mammography and computed tomography (CT), as well as functional imaging methods like single photon emission computed tomography (SPECT).

Chapter 5 – In recent years, Electrical Impedance Tomography (EIT)[1] has been used as a technique that could help health professionals to observe some human body structure behavior. Nowadays, Being EIT a non-invasive, non-radiating, non-ionizing and inexpensive methodology, it has been extensively studied inclinical diagnosis [4], biomedical engineering [5] and biotechnology [6]. Attempts are also being made to develop a better medical EIT system for different clinical investigations and long time patient monitoring. Nowadays, applications do not care about image quality, because these applications are overworking lungs, heart blood flux and, in these situations, there are not important in determining a good image when reconstructed. In spite of that and how EIT is a low cost and a non-invasive technique [4], ones intend to use it for other medical approaches in order to provide a better image reconstruction quality. Although acquisition is reasonably simple, reconstruction EIT images is computationally a hardtask, consisting in a numerical solution of Laplace's equationon specific grid of domain elements, using Finite Element Method (FEM), Finite Differences Method (FDM) and soon [12] [13] [14]. Also, image quality could be improved by a misfit of calculated and measured data in their construction process, creating an error projection approach, called Projection Error-based Regularization.

Chapter 6 - Positron Emission Tomography (PET) is at present the only method affording three-dimensional regional quantitation of various physiological, functional and molecular variables in man. Making use of tracers labelled with short lived positron emitting radio-nuclides and coincidence detection of annihilation radiation state of the art technology and advanced computing systems permit quantitative imaging of voluminous organs within one session. By 3-D data acquisition the distribution of small tracer amounts in the brain can be measured with a spatial resolution of down to 2 mm and values of various metabolic, functional and molecular parameters can be calculated applying kinetic and parametric analysis. Over the last 30 years PET has gained importance as a clinical diagnostic procedure yielding information on pathophysiologic mechanisms in various brain diseases. This method has also been used extensively as a tool of functional neuroanatomy when changes of metabolic or perfusional patterns were studied during various stimulations or task performances in healthy subjects or patients with localized brain lesions. This approach was especially successful in the study of language, which as a complex brain function is based on the interplay of a distributed network in which partial functions are executed in various centres, which are hierarchically organized and lateralized into the dominant hemisphere. Following local brain lesions different language domains are impaired causing the various types of aphasia. Changes in the interactions within the functional network of language are important for the type of aphasia and for the capacity for recovery, e.g. after stroke. In this context, studies of activation patterns during speech tasks in the course after stroke could be used to predict extent of recovery, could demonstrate effects of supportive therapy and may be helpful in the development of procedures, e.g. cortical stimulation, for suppression of interfering or for enhancing compensatory effects in rehabilitation.

Chapter 7 - Functional magnetic resonance imaging (fMRI) is a noninvasive imaging technique that is able to detect hemodynamic changes associated with neuronal activity in vivo. In the past decade, it has been used extensively for mapping functional neuroanatomy in basic neuroscience and clinical applications. A typical fMRI study includes acquisition of a time series of images (during which the subject is instructed to perform certain tasks) and offline processing and analysis of the image series. In real-time fMRI (rtfMRI), however, image processing and analysis start shortly after the beginning of the scan and then follow the image acquisition procedure as closely as possible. Real-time fMRI provides not only a useful tool for effective quality assurance of fMRI studies, but also opportunities for designing functional examinations with interactive controls and feedback. In this chapter, we describe the basic concept and technical solution of rtfMRI, with a focus on a technique that we have recently developed and implemented on a Siemens 3T MRI scanner. We then demonstrate potential applications of rtfMRI techniques for neurofeedback and motion artifact reduction. In particular, we present a novel method of voluntary head-motion suppression using the feedback of the subject's own motion information in real time. This method was tested and the possible influence on the performance of tasks in fMRI study was assessed utilizing a commonly used working memory task.

Our experiments showed that significant suppression of head motion was achieved consistently while the influence on the performance of task and the interference to brain activation could be minimized by careful design of the feedback system.

In: Medical Imaging
Editors: M. D'Elia and A. Madaffari

ISBN: 978-1-62081-049-1

Chapter 1

UTILITY OF WHOLE-BODY FLUORINE-18-FLUORODEOXYGLUCOSE POSITRON EMISSION TOMOGRAPHY IN PATIENTS WITH LARGE-VESSEL VASCULITIS

Giorgio Treglia**, Maria Vittoria Mattoli, Silvia Taralli and Alessandro Giordano

Institute of Nuclear Medicine, Department of Bioimaging and Radiological Sciences, Catholic University of the Sacred Heart, Rome, Italy

ABSTRACT

Objective: To review the emerging role of positron emission tomography (PET) and positron emission tomography/computed tomography (PET/CT) with Fluorine-18-fluorodeoxyglucose (FDG) in patients with large-vessel vasculitis (LVV).

Methods: A literature search of published studies regarding whole-body FDG-PET and PET/CT in patients with LVV was performed.

Results: Main findings of the scientific literature are reported and discussed.

---

* Corresponding Author and reprints requests: Dr. Giorgio Treglia, Institute of Nuclear Medicine, Catholic University of the Sacred Heart Address: Largo Gemelli,8; City: Rome (Italy); Zip code: 00168. Email address: giorgiomednuc@libero.it. fax number: +39063013745 telephone: 390630154978

Conclusions: FDG-PET and PET/CT are useful imaging methods in the initial diagnosis, in the assessment of activity and extent of disease in patients with LVV. The correlation between FDG-PET findings and serological levels of inflammatory markers as well as the usefulness of FDG-PET and PET/CT in evaluating treatment response remain unclear; it appears that there is a superiority of FDG-PET and PET/CT over conventional imaging methods in the diagnosis of LVV, but not in assessing disease activity under immunosuppressive treatment, in predicting relapse or in evaluating vascular complications.

Keywords: Positron emission tomography, ^{18}F- fluorodeoxyglucose, PET/CT, vasculitis, aortitis.

INTRODUCTION

Large-vessel vasculitis (LVV) can be clinically diagnosed and classified according to specific criteria [1-3]. Early diagnosis and assessment of extent of LVV are crucial factors for adequate therapeutic measures. LVV diagnosis is often difficult due to the absence of specific symptoms and signs and the limited specificity of the available biochemical tests. Since morphological imaging techniques such as angiography, computed tomography (CT), magnetic resonance imaging (MRI) and ultrasonography (US) show anatomical changes, the inflammation of the vessel wall cannot be detected in an early phase due to the lack of substantial anatomical changes at this time. It is also difficult to distinguish active inflammatory lesions from residual anatomical changes due to previous inflammation [4,5].

Fluorine-18-fluorodeoxyglucose positron emission tomography (FDG-PET) is a functional non-invasive technique which has become an established tool in oncology [6]. Moreover, this imaging technique has a promising role in the field of inflammatory diseases [4,5,7]. FDG, a glucose analogue, accumulates in cells with increased glycolysis which occurs not exclusively in neoplastic cells. Even lesions with high concentration of activated inflammatory cells show increased FDG uptake. FDG-PET may therefore be a valuable imaging technique for evaluating the metabolic activity of the vessel wall in both the diagnosis and follow-up of patients with LVV [4-7].

Several studies have shown the role of whole-body FDG-PET and PET/CT in patients with LVV, and a recent meta-analysis evaluated the diagnostic performance of FDG-PET in patients with giant cell arteritis (GCA) [8]. A review of relevant published data about FDG-PET and PET/CT in LVV, including patients with GCA, Takayasu arteritis (TA), polymyalgia rheumatica (PMR) and retroperitoneal fibrosis (RF) was performed.

METHODS

A comprehensive computer literature search was conducted in order to find relevant published articles on the role of FDG-PET in LVV; the search was updated until April 2011. The main findings of the literature were reported and discussed.

RESULTS

Thirty-two articles [5,9-39] were reported and discussed included in this review.

1) Role of FDG-PET and PET/CT in the Management of Patients with Giant Cell Arteritis (GCA) and Polymyalgia Rheumatica (PMR)

Contribution of FDG-PET in the Diagnosis, Assessment of Disease Activity, Extent of Disease and Response to Treatment

First of all, Blockmans et al. [9] investigated the role of FDG-PET in the diagnosis of GCA and PMR. A total of 4/6 patients with GCA and 4/5 patients with PMR showed increased FDG uptake in the thoracic vessels compared to 1/23 controls ($p<0.001$). FDG-PET was also able to detect the involvement of the large vessels of the legs in these patients. The Authors concluded that FDG-PET may diagnose LVV and accurately assess the extent of disease [9].

In 2000, the same Authors [10] analyzed a larger group of LVV patients and confirmed that FDG uptake of the large thoracic arteries was significantly more common in GCA or PMR patients (14/25) than in controls (1/44; $p<0.0001$). Vascular FDG uptake in the legs was seen in 16/25 patients with GCA and PMR and in 10/44 controls, respectively ($p<0.001$). There were no significant differences in erythrocyte sedimentation rate (ESR) or C-reactive protein (CRP) levels between LVV patients with or without vascular FDG uptake. Thoracic vascular FDG uptake had a sensitivity for the diagnosis of

GCA or PMR of 56%, a specificity of 98%, a positive predictive value (PPV) of 93% and a negative predictive value (NPV) of 80%. Vascular FDG uptake in the legs had a sensitivity of 64%, but a specificity of 77%. These findings suggested that FDG-PET is a useful tool for evaluating patients with atypical presentations of GCA or PMR [10].

In 2003, Bleeker-Rovers et al. [5] demonstrated that FDG-PET is a useful imaging technique in diagnosing and determining the extent of various forms of vasculitis. FDG-PET was performed in eight patients with LVV (five GCA, two PMR, one TA), six patients with other vasculitis and three patients with other vascular disease. FDG-PET showed a PPV of 100% and a NPV of 82% in the diagnosis of vasculitis [5].

In their preliminary study, de Leeuw et al. [16] found that FDG-PET was a valuable tool in assessing disease activity during follow-up and in evaluating treatment response. The Authors underlined that FDG-PET and morphological imaging (such as angiography) might complement each other, as some discrepancies between these methods were found; in fact, FDG-PET may show inflammatory changes while the morphological imaging is still normal. Conversely, after progression to the late phase of the disease with stenoses and occlusions, inflammation may disappear and FDG-PET might not show the irreversible anatomical changes seen on morphological imaging [16].

In 2005, Walter et al. [20] investigated the role of FDG-PET in the diagnosis of LVV, in assessing disease activity and extent of disease in 26 patients. FDG-PET revealed abnormal findings in 18/26 patients, showing an overall sensitivity of 60%, a specificity of 99.8%, a PPV of 99.7%, a NPV of 67.9%. Increased vascular FDG uptake was significantly correlated with both CRP and ESR levels (p=0.002 and 0.007, respectively). FDG-PET confirmed the diagnosis of extensive disease in six patients and limited disease (only aortic involvement) in 12 patients; additionally, in eight cases the diagnosis of limited disease was upgraded to extensive disease based on FDG-PET findings. PET scans performed in four patients after immunosuppressive treatment showed a marked reduction of disease activity and extension of disease, in agreement with the clinical improvement and the decrease of ESR and CRP levels. These findings demonstrated that FDG-PET is highly effective in assessing the activity and the extent of LVV [20].

In 2008, Janssen et al. confirmed that FDG-PET is both a sensitive and a specific test for diagnosis of GCA: in 9/11 patients evaluated, the diagnosis of GCA was supported by a positive FDG-PET scan, thus suggesting an important role for FDG-PET in the diagnostic work-up of GCA [28].

In the same year, Bruschi et al. [29] evaluated the predictive value of clinical and biochemical features compared to FDG-PET in the diagnostic work-up of 25 patients with LVV. All patients were stratified according to clinical manifestations, serological levels of inflammatory markers and steroid therapy. Both clinical and biochemical features showed low correlation with FDG-PET findings. A negative correlation between steroid dose and number of scans suggestive for LVV has been observed. The Authors concluded that FDG-PET represents a useful diagnostic tool in early stages of LVV and a powerful instrument to follow the treatment response [29].

Role of FDG-PET in Predicting Relapse and Aortic Complications

In 2006, Blockmans et al. [23] evaluated 35 patients with GCA at diagnosis, during steroid treatment and at time of relapse in order to assess whether FDG-PET may predict the relapse of GCA. At diagnosis, abnormal vascular FDG uptake was observed in 29 patients (83%), especially in the subclavian arteries (74%), but also in the aorta (>50%) and up to the femoral arteries (37%). Vascular FDG uptake was reduced at FDG-PET scan performed after three months ($p<0.0005$), but was not further decreased at six month follow-up. The patients who relapsed had similar FDG uptake reductions between the baseline and the follow-up PET scan compared with the patients who did not relapse. The Authors concluded that: 1) increased FDG uptake of the large vessels is a sensitive marker for GCA; 2) FDG-PET does not predict the relapse of GCA [23].

In 2007, the same Authors [24] evaluated FDG uptake in different vascular regions and in the large joints of 35 patients with isolated PMR before and after treatment with steroids, and investigated whether there is a correlation between FDG-PET findings and risk of relapse. At diagnosis, abnormal vascular FDG uptake was noted in 11 patients (31%), predominantly on the subclavian arteries. FDG uptake of the shoulders was observed in 94% of patients, of the hips and spinous processes of the vertebrae in 89% and 51% of patients, respectively. The intensity of vascular FDG uptake did not correlate with the risk of relapse. These findings demonstrated that: 1) only one third of the patients with isolated PMR show abnormal vascular FDG uptake, especially in the subclavian arteries; 2) most PMR patients have inflammation of shoulders and hips; 3) FDG-PET findings in patients with PMR do not correlate with the risk of relapse [24].

Since GCA is associated with an increased risk of developing thoracic aortic aneurysms, Blockmans et al. [26] investigated whether there was a correlation between the extent of vascular FDG uptake during the acute phase of GCA and the aortic diameter measured on CT scan at late follow-up. Forty-six patients with GCA who had an increased aortic FDG uptake at diagnosis, had a significantly larger diameter of the ascending and descending aorta and a significantly larger volume of the thoracic aorta at late follow-up (mean: 46.7 months). The Authors concluded that, at diagnosis, GCA patients with abnormal aortic FDG uptake may be more prone to develop thoracic aortic aneurysms than GCA patients without abnormal aortic FDG uptake [26].

Comparison between FDG-PET and MRI in the Diagnosis and Monitoring of Disease Activity during Immunosuppressive Therapy

In 2003, Meller et al. [11] compared FDG-PET with MRI in 15 patients with LVV, at baseline and during immunosuppressive therapy. At baseline, abnormal FDG uptake was observed in 59/104 (56%) vascular regions evaluated. Seven follow-up FDG-PET scans were performed in six patients: 24/30 (80%) vascular regions showed normalization of FDG uptake in agreement with the clinical improvement and the normalization of the inflammatory markers. Of 76 vascular regions studied with PET, 41 (53%) showed vasculitis on MRI and 47 regions were concordantly positive or negative on both modalities. Eleven vascular regions resulted positive only on MRI while 18 were positive exclusively on PET. MRI was performed during follow-up in six patients showing an improvement in 2/17 vascular regions. These findings demonstrated that FDG-PET is a valuable tool in the early diagnosis of LVV; the results of FDG-PET and MRI in this setting were comparable, but FDG-PET identified more vascular regions involved than MRI. Furthermore, FDG-PET seems to be more reliable than MRI in monitoring disease activity during immunosuppressive therapy [11].

In 2004, Scheel et al. [15] correlated FDG-PET and MRI findings with clinical course and serum levels of inflammatory markers in 8 patients with LVV. At baseline, 20/24 vascular regions were positive on FDG-PET and 15/21 on MRI. After treatment with corticosteroids, 11/20 (55%) vascular regions showed normalization of FDG uptake during follow-up, correlating with clinical improvement and with normalization of the inflammatory markers. Conversely, 14/15 initially affected vascular regions were unchanged on follow-up MRI scans. These findings confirmed that FDG-PET and MRI are both effective techniques for detecting early LVV, but FDG-PET is more reliable than MRI in evaluating treatment response [15].

In 2008, Both et al. [27] compared MRI with FDG-PET for the assessment of disease activity in 25 patients with complicated GCA despite immunosuppressive therapy. Active disease was detected by MRI and FDG-

PET in 22 and 20 patients, respectively. While serological and clinical findings correlated significantly, there was no concordance with MRI findings and a not significant correlation between FDG-PET and CRP (p=0.136), ESR (p=0.320) and clinical findings (p=0.221). The Authors concluded that MRI and FDG-PET are unreliable for assessing large-vessel inflammation in patients with complicated GCA during immunosuppressive therapy [27].

Comparison between FDG-PET and US in the Diagnosis of GCA

In 2004, Brodmann et al. [13] evaluated 22 GCA patients with US and FDG-PET before treatment with corticosteroids. Six patients had involvement of both large arteries and temporal arteries; five patients show the exclusive involvement of the large arteries and the remaining 11 patients showed the exclusive involvement of the temporal arteries. All patients with suggestive findings of GCA of the large vessels on US showed increased FDG uptake in the same vessels. When positive US was limited to the temporal arteries, FDG-PET was completely negative. The Authors concluded that FDG-PET is not suitable for the diagnosis of temporal arteritis and therefore cannot replace invasive biopsy. FDG-PET is suitable to demonstrate GCA of large arteries [13].

Recently, Pfadenhauer et al. [38] evaluated the ability of FDG-PET to detect active GCA of the extracerebral vertebral artery (VA) compared to clinical, US and biopsy findings in 46 patients. Fifteen of the 46 (33%) GCA patients had abnormal FDG uptake of the VA. In 2/15 patients (4%) increased FDG uptake of a single VA was the only PET abnormality while in 13/15 patients a concomitant increased FDG uptake of the large arteries was observed. FDG-PET was superior to US for the detection of active GCA, including VA involvement. A strong correlation between PET abnormalities in VA and clinical abnormalities was observed in 2/3 of patients. Abnormal vascular FDG uptake was detectable in five patients despite the glucocorticoid treatment. These findings demonstrated that abnormal FDG uptake of the VA can be an early and isolated finding of active GCA and it can be detected in some cases despite steroid treatment [38].

Value of Semi-Quantitative PET Analysis

In 2004, Moosig et al. [14] visually and semi-quantitatively assessed FDG uptake of the large vessels in 13 untreated patients with PMR, and compared these data with the serological levels of the inflammatory markers. Visually, 12/13 patients showed an increased FDG uptake of the aorta or its major branches. By semi-quantitative analysis, using region of interest placed on the vascular regions and on the lung (considered as background region), FDG uptake was significantly increased in PMR patients; the regions which best discriminated between active PMR and controls were the subclavian and external carotid arteries. In eight patients who underwent follow-up PET, FDG uptake was significantly reduced. In active PMR, FDG uptake was significantly related to CRP (r=0.8) and ESR (r=0.79) levels. The Authors concluded that increased FDG uptake of the large vessels and a strong correlation between FDG uptake and inflammatory markers are suggestive findings of LVV. Furthermore, semi-quantitative PET analysis appears to be a sensitive tool for LVV detection [14].

In 2008 [30], Hautzel et al. performed a semi-quantitative analysis calculating the aortic to liver FDG uptake ratio in a group of 18 GCA patients and in a control group. A receiver operating characteristic (ROC) analysis revealed a sensitivity of 88.9%, a specificity of 95.1%, and an accuracy of 94.4%. for a cutoff aorta-to-liver FDG uptake ratio of 1.0. The Authors concluded that PET semi-quantitative analysis using aorta to liver FDG uptake ratio is a reliable, investigator-independent indicator of GCA [30].

Recently, Lehmann et al. [37] evaluated the diagnostic accuracy of FDG-PET in LVV, using a visual and a semi-quantitative analysis (by using the standardized uptake value, SUV). Twenty LVV patients and 20 controls were evaluated. The specificity of visual analysis was 80% and the sensitivity was 65%, yielding an overall diagnostic accuracy of 72%. FDG uptake of the subclavian regions was significantly higher in LVV than in control patients (p=0.016). PET findings were reproducible and observer-independent. ROC analysis revealed the highest sensitivity of 90% and specificity of 45% for a maximum SUV cutoff point of 1.78. The Authors concluded that LVV diagnosis should consider the clinical context and cannot be exclusively based on FDG-PET findings [37].

The Potential Added Value of Hybrid PET/CT

In 2008, Henes et al. [31] determined the value of FDG-PET/CT for the diagnosis and re-evaluation of LVV in 13 patients. FDG-PET/CT revealed active LVV despite nearly normal ESR and CRP levels in some patients. A long segmental increased FDG uptake of the vessel wall was indicative of vascular inflammation. The aortic arch was involved in all patients with active disease (n=12). In the complementary CT scans, vascular stenosis was found in 8/13 patients. The Authors concluded that:1) ESR and CRP levels are not sufficient to evaluate disease activity in LVV; 2) PET/CT allows the evaluation of disease activity and vessel morphology as well as the localization of the inflammatory sites in the same session [31].

Recently, Papathanasiou et al. [39] investigated the diagnostic performance of FDG-PET/CT in 78 patients with suspected LVV. According to clinical diagnosis, patients were classified into three groups: a) steroid-naive LVV (16 patients), b) LVV on steroid treatment (18 patients) and c) no evidence of LVV (44 patients). FDG-PET/CT was positive in patients with steroid-naive LVV and in these patients FDG vascular uptake was significantly higher than in other groups ($p<0.05$). The thoracic aorta, carotid and subclavian arteries were most frequently involved. A significant positive association ($p<0.05$) was found between FDG uptake of the thoracic aorta and inflammatory markers in LVV patients. The patients on steroid treatment showed lower FDG vascular uptake than steroid-naive patients. These findings demonstrated that FDG-PET/CT can detect the extent and activity of LVV in untreated patients but it is unreliable for LVV diagnosis in patients on steroid treatment [39].

2) Role of FDG-PET and PET/CT in Patients with TA

In 2003, Meller et al. [12] compared FDG-PET and MRI in five patients with TA. Abnormal FDG uptake in the aortic wall was noted in all patients; 26/34 (76%) vascular regions studied by FDG-PET showed increased FDG uptake. Conversely, 9/28 (32%) vascular regions studied by MRI showed abnormal findings suggestive of vasculitis. The Authors concluded that: 1) FDG-PET is a suitable whole-body imaging method in the diagnosis of TA; 2) MRI remains indispensable in the exact determination of the morphological changes and in the documentation of complications such as stenosis, aneurysms and occlusions [12].

In 2004, Andrews et al. [17] confirmed that FDG-PET and MRI provide useful information for early diagnosis and management of TA. Such techniques allowed a more accurate assessment of treatment response than conventional clinical assessment and/or angiography in six patients evaluated [17].

In the same year, Webb et al. [18] assessed the role of FDG-PET in 18 patients with TA, reporting a sensitivity of 92%, a specificity of 100%, a NPV of 85% and a PPV of 100% in the assessment of active TA compared with the combined assessment of disease activity based on symptoms, biochemical markers and angiography findings. The predominant FDG uptake pattern in positive FDG-PET scans was linear and continuous. Follow-up FDG-PET scan performed in eight patients showed agreement with clinical assessment of disease activity. The Authors found that FDG-PET is more likely to be positive when the inflammatory markers are higher. These findings suggested that FDG-PET can be used to diagnose early disease, to detect active disease and to monitor the effectiveness of treatment in patients with TA [18].

In 2005, Kobayashi et al. [19] evaluated the ability of FDG-PET co-registered with enhanced CT to assess the disease activity in 14 patients with TA. A semi-quantitative analysis by using the SUV was performed. PET showed intense FDG uptake (SUV>2.7) of the vascular wall of the large vessels in 2/11 cases of active TA. The other nine patients with active TA showed weak FDG vascular uptake (2.3>SUV>1.2). No significant FDG uptake was observed in three patients with inactive disease (SUV<1.2) and controls (SUV<1.3). Given the cutoff SUV of 1.3, the sensitivity of FDG-PET in detecting active TA was 90.9% and the specificity was 88.8%. FDG-PET co-registered with enhanced CT localized inflammation of the aortic wall of TA patients that could not otherwise be morphologically identified. Finally, vascular FDG uptake resolved with steroid therapy in two active cases; the disappearance of FDG uptake did not correlate with the serological levels of inflammatory markers. These findings demonstrated that FDG-PET images co-registered with enhanced CT images are useful in assessing the disease activity in patients with TA [19].

In 2009, Arnaud et al. [32] investigated the value of FDG-PET/CT in assessing the disease activity of 28 TA patients, by comparing PET findings with clinical, serological and MRI findings. The pattern of vascular FDG uptake in positive PET scans was diffuse (73%), segmental (20%), or focal (13%). There was a not significant association between clinically active disease and FDG vascular uptake (p=0.08). PET scans obtained for assessment of clinically active disease had a sensitivity of 69.2%, a specificity of 33.3%, a PPV of 33.3%, and a NPV of 69.2%. No statistical association between serological levels of inflammatory markers and intensity of FDG vascular uptake was found. There was a not significant association between FDG vascular uptake and the presence of vascular wall thickening, gadolinium uptake, or the presence of vascular wall edema on MRI. These findings demonstrated the absence of a significant association between FDG vascular uptake and clinical, serological or MRI assessment of disease activity in TA patients [32].

Also Lee et al. [33] evaluated the usefulness of FDG-PET/CT in detecting active disease in 32 patients with TA. Ten patients had active lesions on FDG-

PET/CT showing high-grade, linear FDG uptake along the aortic wall. Compared with clinical disease activity criteria, FDG-PET/CT had a sensitivity of 78% and a specificity of 87%. ESR and CRP levels were significantly higher in PET positive than in PET negative patients. There was a not significant difference in the proportion of positive PET scans according to the use of immunosuppressive therapy. The Authors concluded that the sensitivity of FDG-PET/CT for detecting active disease was higher in TA patients with higher serological levels of inflammatory markers. The specificity of FDG-PET/CT was also high. However, in interpreting these findings, it should be kept in mind that the clinical disease activity criteria have low sensitivity in detecting pathologically proven active disease [33].

Recently, Bertagna et al. [34] evaluated eight patients with TA by FDG-PET/CT before and after corticosteroid treatment, demonstrating that this method is an accurate tool for establishing the diagnosis of TA, for evaluating disease extension and for monitoring therapy in conjunction with clinical and biochemical findings [34].

3) Role of FDG-PET in Patients with Chronic Periaortitis and Retroperitoneal Fibrosis

CP is characterized by a fibro-inflammatory reaction that extends from the adventitia of the abdominal aorta and common iliac arteries into the retroperitoneum, often leading to the involvement of adjacent structures (ureters, inferior vena cava). Three main entities are included: idiopathic retroperitoneal fibrosis (IRF), perianeurysmal retroperitoneal fibrosis (PRF), and inflammatory abdominal aortic aneurysms (IAAA). In patients with CP, FDG-PET shows the presence of a LVV involving abdominal aorta and common iliac arteries, which in some patients is also extended to the thoracic aorta and/or its branches, as demonstrated by Salvarani et al. [21].

Nakajo et al. confirmed that FDG-PET and PET/CT are useful tools for evaluating disease activity and extent of RF, but these methods fail to differentiate between malignancy and RF [25].

Vaglio et al [22] used FDG-PET to evaluate the metabolic activity of residual masses at CT scan after immunosuppressive treatment in patients with RF. Six of seven patients evaluated had no abnormal FDG uptake in the residual mass and the seventh showed only moderate aorto-iliac FDG uptake. During the follow-up, none of the patients showed clinical, serological or radiological signs of disease relapse. These findings suggest that FDG-PET is a sensitive mean to evaluate metabolic activity of residual masses in IRF patients in clinical remission with detectable masses at CT scans [22].

Recently, Piccoli et al. [35] supported the use of FDG-PET/CT not only for the diagnostic work-up but also in the follow-up of patients with RF, in order to tailor medical and surgical approaches. In particular, the comparison between the FDG-PET scans acquired during the diagnostic work-up and during follow-up may be useful to identify the best time for a safe removal of the renal stents and to schedule for tapering of immunosuppressive therapy, crucial issues to reduce morbidity and improve the quality of life of RF patients [35].

At last, Jansen et al. [36] evaluated whether FDG-PET was useful in the diagnostic and therapeutic evaluation of patients with RF treated with tamoxifen. At baseline, FDG-PET was positive in 20/26 patients. Patients with a positive FDG-PET scan had higher CRP level ($p=0.02$) and larger mass size at CT scan ($p=0.01$) compared with patients with a negative FDG-PET scan. FDG uptake decreased following treatment, in agreement with ESR reduction ($p<0.001$), but not with CT-documented mass regression. These findings demonstrated that: 1) FDG-PET may be useful to evaluate the severity and the extent of RF, 2) FDG-PET may be a valuable tool in assessing disease activity during or after treatment in patients with normal inflammatory markers levels and stable residual mass on repeated CT scans [36].

Conclusion

From this review on the role of FDG-PET and PET/CT in patients with LVV we are led to conclude that:

1) FDG-PET and PET/CT are useful imaging methods in the early diagnosis, in the assessment of activity and extent of the disease;
2) the correlation between FDG-PET findings and serological levels of inflammatory markers (at diagnosis and under immunosuppressive treatment) as well as the usefulness of FDG-PET and PET/CT in evaluating treatment response remain unclear issues which need to be further investigated;
3) it appears that there is a superiority of FDG-PET and PET/CT over conventional imaging methods (such as US or MRI) in the diagnosis of LVV, but not in assessing disease activity under immuno-suppressive treatment, in predicting relapse or in evaluating vascular

complications; further studies should focus on the comparison of FDG-PET/CT with US and MRI;

4) given the heterogeneity among the various studies for PET analysis and diagnostic criteria, a standardization of the technique is required, in order to achieve reproducible and inter-observer independent results.

References

[1] Arend WP, Michel BA, Bloch DA, Hunder GG, Calabrese LH, Edworthy SM et al. The American College of Rheumatology 1990 criteria for the classification of Takayasu arteritis. *Arthritis. Rheum.*, 1990;33:1129-34.

[2] Hunder GG, Bloch DA, Michel BA, Stevens MB, Arend WP, Calabrese LH et al. The American College of Rheumatology 1990 criteria for the classification of giant cell arteritis. *Arthritis. Rheum.*, 1990;33:1122-8.

[3] Healey LA. Long-term follow-up of polymyalgia rheumatica: evidence for synovitis. *Semin. Arthritis. Rheum.*, 1984;13:322-8.

[4] Gotthardt M, Bleeker-Rovers CP, Boerman OC, Oyen WJ. Imaging of inflammation by PET, conventional scintigraphy, and other imaging techniques. *J. Nucl. Med.*, 2010;51:1937-49.

[5] Bleeker-Rovers CP, Bredie SJ, van der Meer JW, Corstens FH, Oyen WJ. F-18-fluorodeoxyglucose positron emission tomography in diagnosis and follow-up of patients with different types of vasculitis. *Neth. J. Med.*, 2003;61:323-9.

[6] Treglia G, Cason E, Fagioli G. Recent applications of nuclear medicine in diagnostics - first part. *Ital. J. Med.*, 2010; 4:84-91.

[7] Treglia G, Cason E, Fagioli G. Recent applications of nuclear medicine in diagnostics - second part. *Ital. J. Med.*, 2010; 4:159-166.

[8] Besson FL, Parienti JJ, Bienvenu B, Prior JO, Costo S, Bouvard G et al. Diagnostic performance of (18)F-fluorodeoxyglucose positron emission tomography in giant cell arteritis: a systematic review and meta-analysis. *Eu.r J. Nucl. Med. Mol. Imaging*, 2011; 38;1764-72.

[9] Blockmans D, Maes A, Stroobants S, Nuyts J, Bormans G, Knockaert D et al. New arguments for a vasculitic nature of polymyalgia rheumatica using positron emission tomography. *Rheumatology*, 1999;38:444-7.

[10] Blockmans D, Stroobants S, Maes A, Mortelmans L. Positron emission tomography in giant cell arteritis and polymyalgia rheumatica: evidence for inflammation of the aortic arch. *Am. J. Med.*, 2000;108:246-9.

[11] Meller J, Strutz F, Siefker U, Scheel A, Sahlmann CO, Lehmann K et al. Early diagnosis and follow-up of aortitis with [(18)F]FDG PET and MRI. *Eur. J. Nucl. Med. Mol. Imaging*, 2003;30:730-6.

[12] Meller J, Grabbe E, Becker W, Vosshenrich R. Value of F-18 FDG hybrid camera PET and MRI in early takayasu aortitis. *Eur. Radiol.*, 2003;13:400-5.

[13] Brodmann M, Lipp RW, Passath A, Seinost G, Pabst E, Pilger E. The role of 2-18F-fluoro-2-deoxy-D-glucose positron emission tomography in the diagnosis of giant cell arteritis of the temporal arteries. *Rheumatology*, 2004;43:241-2.

[14] Moosig F, Czech N, Mehl C, Henze E, Zeuner RA, Kneba M, Schröder JO. Correlation between 18-fluorodeoxyglucose accumulation in large vessels and serological markers of inflammation in polymyalgia rheumatica: a quantitative PET study. *Ann. Rheum. Dis.*, 2004;63:870-3.

[15] Scheel AK, Meller J, Vosshenrich R, Kohlhoff E, Siefker U, Müller GA, Strutz F. Diagnosis and follow up of aortitis in the elderly. *Ann. Rheum. Dis.*, 2004;63:1507-10.

[16] de Leeuw K, Bijl M, Jager PL. Additional value of positron emission tomography in diagnosis and follow-up of patients with large vessel vasculitides. *Clin. Exp. Rheumatol.*, 2004;22(6 Suppl 36):S21-6.

[17] Andrews J, Al-Nahhas A, Pennell DJ, Hossain MS, Davies KA, Haskard DO, Mason JC. Non-invasive imaging in the diagnosis and management of Takayasu's arteritis. *Ann. Rheum. Dis.,* 2004;63:995-1000.

[18] Webb M, Chambers A, Al-Nahhas A, Mason JC, Maudlin L, Rahman L, Frank J. The role of 18F-FDG PET in characterising disease activity in Takayasu arteritis. *Eur. J. Nucl. Med. Mol. Imaging*, 2004; 31:627-34.

[19] Kobayashi Y, Ishii K, Oda K, Nariai T, Tanaka Y, Ishiwata K, Numano F. Aortic wall inflammation due to Takayasu arteritis imaged with 18F-FDG PET coregistered with enhanced CT. *J. Nucl. Med.,* 2005;46:917-22.

[20] Walter MA, Melzer RA, Schindler C, Müller-Brand J, Tyndall A, Nitzsche EU. The value of [18F]FDG-PET in the diagnosis of large-vessel vasculitis and the assessment of activity and extent of disease. Eur. *J. Nucl. Med. Mol. Imaging*, 2005;32:674-81.

[21] Salvarani C, Pipitone N, Versari A, Vaglio A, Serafini D, Bajocchi G et al. Positron emission tomography (PET): evaluation of chronic periaortitis. *Arthritis Rheum.*, 2005;53:298-303.

[22] Vaglio A, Greco P, Versari A, Filice A, Cobelli R, Manenti L et al. Post-treatment residual tissue in idiopathic retroperitoneal fibrosis: active residual disease or silent "scar" ? A study using 18F-fluorodeoxyglucose positron emission tomography. *Clin. Exp. Rheumatol.*, 2005;23:231-4.

[23] Blockmans D, de Ceuninck L, Vanderschueren S, Knockaert D, Mortelmans L, Bobbaers H. Repetitive 18F-fluorodeoxyglucose positron emission tomography in giant cell arteritis: a prospective study in 35 patients. *Arthritis Rheum.*, 2006;55:131-7.

[24] Blockmans D, de Ceuninck L, Vanderschueren S, Knockaert D, Mortelmans L, Bobbaers H. Repetitive 18F-fluorodeoxyglucose positron emission tomography in isolated polymyalgia rheumatica: a prospective study of 35 patients. *Rheumatology*, 2006;55:131-7.

[25] Nakajo M, Jinnouchi S, Tanabe H, Tateno R, Nakajo M. 18F-fluorodeoxyglucose positron emission tomography features of idiopathic retroperitoneal fibrosis. *J. Comput. Assist. Tomogr.*, 2007; 31:539-43.

[26] Blockmans D, Coudyzer W, Vanderschueren S, Stroobants S, Loeckx D, Heye S et al. Relationship between fluorodeoxyglucose uptake in the large vessels and late aortic diameter in giant cell arteritis. *Rheumatology*, 2008;47:1179-84.

[27] Both M, Ahmadi-Simab K, Reuter M, Dourvos O, Fritzer E, Ullrich S et al. MRI and FDG-PET in the assessment of inflammatory aortic arch syndrome in complicated courses of giant cell arteritis. *Ann. Rheum. Dis.*, 2008;67:1030-3.

[28] Janssen SP, Comans EH, Voskuyl AE, Wisselink W, Smulders YM. Giant cell arteritis: heterogeneity in clinical presentation and imaging results. *J. Vasc. Surg.*, 2008;48:1025-31.

[29] Bruschi M, De Leonardis F, Govoni M, Roncali M, Prandini N, La Corte R et al. 18FDG-PET and large vessel vasculitis: preliminary data on 25 patients. *Reumatismo.*, 2008;60:212-6.

[30] Hautzel H, Sander O, Heinzel A, Schneider M, Müller HW. Assessment of large-vessel involvement in giant cell arteritis with 18F-FDG PET: introducing an ROC-analysis-based cutoff ratio. *J. Nucl. Med.,* 2008;49:1107-13.

[31] Henes JC, Müller M, Krieger J, Balletshofer B, Pfannenberg AC, Kanz L, Kötter I. [18F] FDG-PET/CT as a new and sensitive imaging method

for the diagnosis of large vessel vasculitis. *Clin. Exp. Rheumatol.*, 2008;26(3 Suppl 49):S47-52.

[32] Arnaud L, Haroche J, Malek Z, Archambaud F, Gambotti L, Grimon G et al. Is (18)F-fluorodeoxyglucose positron emission tomography scanning a reliable way to assess disease activity in Takayasu arteritis? *Arthritis. Rheum.*, 2009;60:1193-200.

[33] Lee SG, Ryu JS, Kim HO, Oh JS, Kim YG, Lee CK, Yoo B. Evaluation of disease activity using F-18 FDG PET-CT in patients with Takayasu arteritis. *Clin. Nucl. Med.*, 2009;34:749-52.

[34] Bertagna F, Bosio G, Caobelli F, Motta F, Biasiotto G, Giubbini R. Role of 18F-fluorodeoxyglucose positron emission tomography/computed tomography for therapy evaluation of patients with large-vessel vasculitis. *Jpn. J. Radiol.,* 2010;28:199-204.

[35] Piccoli GB, Consiglio V, Arena V, Pelosi E, Anastasios D, Ragni F et al. Positron emission tomography as a tool for the 'tailored' management of retroperitoneal fibrosis: a nephro-urological experience. *Nephrol. Dial. Transplant.*, 2010;25:2603-10.

[36] Jansen I, Hendriksz TR, Han SH, Huiskes AW, van Bommel EF. (18)F-fluorodeoxyglucose position emission tomography (FDG-PET) for monitoring disease activity and treatment response in idiopathic retroperitoneal fibrosis. *Eur. J. Intern. Med.*, 2010;21:216-21.

[37] Lehmann P, Buchtala S, Achajew N, Haerle P, Ehrenstein B, Lighvani H et al. 18F-FDG PET as a diagnostic procedure in large vessel vasculitis-a controlled, blinded re-examination of routine PET scans. *Clin. Rheumatol.*, 2011;30:37-42.

[38] Pfadenhauer K, Weinerth J, Hrdina C. Vertebral arteries: a target for FDG-PET imaging in giant cell arteritis? Clinical, ultrasonographic and PET study in 46 patients. *Nuklearmedizin.*, 2011;50:28-32.

[39] Papathanasiou ND, Du Y, Menezes LJ, Al-Muhaideb A, Shastry M, Beynon H, Bomanji JB. 18F-Fluorodeoxyglucose PET/CT in the evaluation of large-vessel vasculitis: diagnostic performance and correlation with clinical and laboratory parameters. *Br. J. Radiol.,* 2011; doi:10.1259/bjr/1642295.

In: Medical Imaging
Editors: M. D'Elia and A. Madaffari
ISBN: 978-1-62081-049-1

Chapter 2

ROBUST REGISTRATION OF HISTOLOGICAL IMAGES: TECHNIQUES AND APPLICATIONS

Wei-Yen Hsu *
Graduate Institute of Biomedical Informatics
Taipei Medical University
Taipei, Taiwan

ABSTRACT

Image registration that is used to reconstruct 3D structure of tissues from a series of images is an important topic in medical image analysis. However, it becomes a difficult challenge for image registration due to a variety of inherent factors, such as color difference and geometry discrepancy. In this chapter, a robust registration algorithm is proposed to automatically reconstruct 3D volume data from histological images. It mainly contains three procedures, including wavelet-based feature extraction, analytic robust point matching (ARPM), and registration refinement by modified Levenberg-Marquardt algorithm (FMLM). The concept that features could exist in multiscale is used to extract true feature points. The ARPM registration algorithm is then proposed to speedily accomplish the registration of two point sets with different size by simultaneously evaluating the spatial correspondence and geometrical transformation. Finally, a FMLM method is used to further refine

---

* Email: shenswy@gmail.com; shen@csie.ncku.edu.tw
Tel: +886-2-27361661 ext. 3350

registration results and achieve subpixel accuracy. The performance of proposed method is evaluated in comparison with several well-known approaches. The results indicate that the proposed method is a robust and fast method in image registration.

Keywords: Medical image registration; Neuro-informatics; Spatial correspondence; Analytic robust point matching; Modified Levenberg-Marquardt algorithm.

1. INTRODUCTION

Image registration is essential in various biomedical fields and has been investigated over the past few decades. It has been applied to many applications, including medical image analysis, 3D reconstruction, surveillance operations, video representation and retrieval, and remote sensing, with different registration techniques and performance requirements (Chakravarty et al., 2006; Cornillie et al., 2008; Fernandez-Gonzalez et al., 2002; Holden, 2008; Lebenberg et al., 2010; Simonetti et al., 2006; Yelnik et al., 2007). It is mainly the process of spatially registering acquired image slices so that corresponding features or pixels on them are consistent in geometry. In biomedical research, image registration is used to unite complementary information to improve visualization of regions of interest for clinical or research purposes. A variety of medical image registration techniques have been presented (DâââAgostino et al., 2006; Gholipour et al., 2007; Zacharaki et al., 2008). A common biomedical problem for image registration is to align all the acquired experimental image sequence into a complete volume. Alignment of biomedical images requires a registration algorithm that will compensate as much as possible for geometric variability among images. Numerous methods accounting for nonlinear differences have been proposed. In general, image registration techniques are classified as feature-based and intensity-based methods.

Intensity-based methods are based on pixel intensities and certain optimized objective functions (Gefen et al., 2008; Klein et al., 2010), while feature-based ones are performed by maximizing a similarity measure computed from the correspondences under the assumption that point correspondences are available in adjacent images (Hsu et al., 2008; Shu and Chung, 2010). In addition, some approaches use deformable models to track a large nonlinear deformation (Droske and Rumpf, 2007; Han et al., 2003). A registration algorithm usually minimizes a cost function that is a combination of an objective function and smoothness constraint (Chetverikov et al., 2005; Foroughi et al., 2006; Loeckx et al., 2010; Walimbe and Shekhar, 2006). There are lots of algorithms that iteratively minimize the surface distance in order to linearly align two regions, such as iterative closest point (ICP) algorithms. In this chapter, we focus on the robust and fast mapping. In other words, in addition to the registration accuracy, the time cost is also considered.

In this chapter, we propose a robust registration method, which consist of multiscale wavelet-based feature extraction, a registration approach based on analytic robust point matching (ARPM), and a refinement procedure of feature-based modified Levenberg-Marquardt algorithm (FMLM), to automatically reconstruct 3D vessels of the rat brains from a series of microscopic images. The ARPM registration algorithm could speedily evaluate the spatial correspondence and geometrical transformation between two point sets with different sizes. It is robust to noise and tolerant to deformation produced from color difference and geometry discrepancy. The FMLM refinement algorithm could further refine registration results and speedily achieve subpixel accuracy owing to its feature-based and nonlinear characteristic. Finally, 3D volume data of the rat brain are reconstructed from a series of microscopic images.

The paper is organized as follows: Section II describes the materials and proposed method in detail. In section III, experimental results and the discussion for the registration of rat brains are presented. Finally, the conclusion is given in Section IV.

2. Materials and Methods

Features may lead to large differences in acquired slices even if they are adjacent due to a variety of inherent factors, such as microscopic optics, mechanism, sensors, and manipulation. Local deformation of slices is frequently occurred in the process of imaging. In addition, there is an obvious change in appearance among slices because they are acquired at different time. It is the reason we propose a robust ARPM-FMLM algorithm to solve the problems. The flowchart of the proposed method is illustrated in Figure 1. It consists of three procedures, multiscale wavelet-based feature extraction, ARPM registration algorithm, and registration refinement with FMLM algorithm.

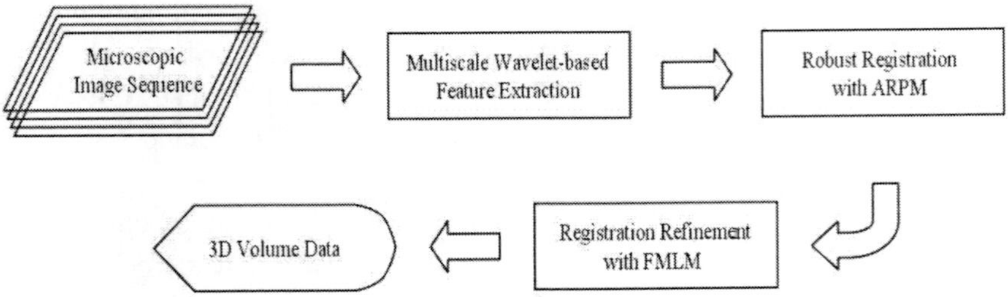

Figure 1. Flowchart of the proposed method. It consists of three procedures, including multiscale wavelet-based feature extraction, robust registration with ARPM, and registration refinement with FMLM.

2.1. Materials

We reconstruct histological volume data from a series of 50μm thick c-Fos immuno-histochemistry-stained histological sections of the rat brain cut. The c-Fos staining is used to enhance the contrast of brain cell bodies to make feature extraction procedure smoothly. There are total 97 slices in the volume data. Each image is acquired from slices in 1392×1040 pixel 24bit RGB format. However, with this instrument frozen tissue is cut with a microtome and the revealed block-face surface imaged. The sequential images are registered by virtue of the accurate repositioning of the tissue. Tissue differentiation is achieved by systemic staining. We focus the efforts on the registration of rat brain images from microscopic image sequences in this chapter.

2.2. Feature Extraction

Feature extraction is the first and crucial step to obtain significant information from acquired images. It has a great influence on the accuracy of feature-based image registration. The important issue for feature extraction is how to extract significant features from the adjacent images, so as to effectively provide the geometrical and photometric information for image registration. Multi-resolution image decomposition is a useful technique for analyzing image information at various scales. Therefore, wavelet-based edge correlation, which had been verified the efficacy in feature extraction in our previous work (Hsu et al., 2008), is used to extract the feature points with strong and consistent responses under different scales within a local area. In other words, feature points usually have larger values on the product of gradient moduli from multiscales, while the noise does not.

Due to the separable characteristic of wavelet transform, we represent 2D wavelet transform as two 1D ones in x and y directions, $\phi^H(x,y) = \frac{\partial S(x,y)}{\partial x}$ and $\phi^V(x,y) = \frac{\partial S(x,y)}{\partial y}$, where H and V stand for the meaning of horizontal and vertical directions, respectively, and $S(x,y)$ is a 2D smoothing function. We denote $\phi_j(x,y) = \frac{1}{2^{2j}}\phi(\frac{x}{2^j},\frac{y}{2^j})$ as a dilation function of $\phi(x,y)$ by a scaling factor j. The gradients $G_j f(x,y)$ of an image $f(x,y)$ in the x and y directions and its modulus $M_j f(x,y)$ at level j are described as follows:

$$M_j f(x,y) = \sqrt{\left| G_j^H f(x,y)\right|^2 + \left| G_j^V f(x,y)\right|^2} \quad (1)$$

where

$$G_j^H f(x,y) = f * \phi_j^H(x,y) = 2^j \cdot \frac{\partial}{\partial x}(f * S_j)(x,y)$$

$$G_j^V f(x,y) = f * \phi_j^V(x,y) = 2^j \cdot \frac{\partial}{\partial y}(f * S_j)(x,y)$$

All the edge points in image $f(x,y)$ at level j is located with local maxima of $M_j f(x,y)$. The edge correlation filters out the noise by a multiscale edge confirmation to detect reliable feature points.

$$C_n(j,x,y) = \prod_{i=0}^{n-1} M_{j+i} f(x,y), \quad (2)$$

where n is the level number, and j is the initial level. We can obtain true feature points by means of edge correlation. Features and noise sometimes coexist in the wavelet domain, but features can usually exist in multiscales while noise can not (Hsieh et al., 1997; Hsu et al., 2008). In this chapter, the observed property is used to distinguish the true feature points from noise.

2.3. Image Registration

The RPM algorithm is first proposed by Chui and Rangarajan (Chui and Rangarajan, 2003). It is a robust method for point-based registration. Following the notation in (Chui and Rangarajan, 2003; Zheng and Doermann, 2006), we describe the proposed ARPM algorithm in detail.

Given two point-sets $\{u_i, i = 1,2,\ldots,H\}$ and $\{v_j, j = 1,2,\ldots,K\}$ extracted from adjacent slices, and the correspondence mapping is denoted by a matrix M consisting of m_{ij}. The entire energy function minimized by the ARPM algorithm is as follows:

$$E(M,T,W) = \sum_{i=1}^{H}\sum_{j=1}^{K} m_{ij}\left\|u_i - v_j T - \phi(v_j)W\right\|^2 - \alpha\sum_{i=1}^{H}\sum_{j=1}^{K} m_{ij} + \beta\sum_{i=1}^{H}\sum_{j=1}^{K} m_{ij}\log m_{ij}$$
$$+ \lambda_1 trace\left[(T-I)^t(T-I)\right] + \lambda_2 trace\left(W^T \Phi W\right) \quad (3)$$

where $m_{ij} \in [0,1]$ and it subjects to $\sum_{i=1}^{H+1} m_{ij} = 1, \quad \forall j \in \{1,2,\ldots,K\}$ and $\sum_{j=1}^{K+1} m_{ij} = 1, \quad \forall i \in \{1,2,\ldots,H\}$, and T and W represent the geometric transformation and warping coefficient matrix, respectively. The size of matrix M is $(H+1)\times(K+1)$ and its inner $H \times K$ portion indicates the correspondence information for two point-sets. If a point u_i corresponds to a point v_j, then the entry m_{ij} of the correspondence matrix M is equal to 1; otherwise, it is assigned to zero. In addition, in order to take the outliers into account so as to still hold the constraints of the row and column summation to one, an additional row and column is appended to the suffix of the correspondence matrix M.

All the components of the energy function are interpreted in turn in the following: The first term $\sum_{i=1}^{H}\sum_{j=1}^{K} m_{ij}\left\|u_i - v_j T - \phi(v_j)W\right\|^2$ is the error term that it describes a corresponding problem by means of the perspective transformation. It is a desirable transformation since the rotation, scaling, translation, and global shear are all taken into account. The second term $\alpha\sum_{i=1}^{H}\sum_{j=1}^{K}m_{ij}$ with the weighting α is used to avoid excessively much null correspondence. If α is large, then fewer points are discarded as outliers. The third term $\beta\sum_{i=1}^{H}\sum_{j=1}^{K}m_{ij}\log m_{ij}$ with the temperature parameter β is an entropy function that it avoids the elements of correspondence matrix M being negatives. The fourth term $\lambda_1 trace\left[(T-I)^t(T-I)\right]$ with the weighting λ_1 is a constraint on the geometric transformation T by means of the penalty on the remainder of subtracting the identity matrix I from the correspondence matrix T. The final term $\lambda_2 trace\left(W^T\Phi W\right)$ with the weighting λ_2 is a constraint on the warping coefficient matrix W by means of the penalty on the warping coefficient matrix W.

As above mentioned, the minimization problem in equation (3) mainly consists of two related sub-problems: the point-sets correspondence and the geometric transformation between two adjacent slices. Given the point-sets correspondence, the geometric transformation can be evaluated by resolving the constrained least-squares problem. Given the geometric transformation, the point-sets correspondence is found and achieved by resolving the linear assignment problem. Inspired by the idea, the algorithm incorporates the update scheme by alternating the update of the correspondence and the transformation parameters while keeping the other fixed, it is expected to jointly improve the two solutions as well as finally converge to the optimal solution.

The registration algorithm mainly consists of two principal steps. It is accomplished by using alternating update scheme. The first step is to update the point-sets correspondence matrix M as well as make sure that M corresponds to the row and column summation constraints all the time by keeping T and W fixed, with its currently evaluated transformation. Afterwards, the solution for correspondence matrix M could be calculated by means of the differentiation of the energy function in equation (3) with respect to m_{ij},

$$m_{ij} = \exp\left(-\frac{\left\| u_i - v_j T - \phi(v_j) W \right\|^2 - \alpha}{\beta} \right) \tag{4}$$

The second step is to update the parameters of geometric transformation T and warping coefficient matrix W with the correspondence matrix M held fixed. We propose an analytic differential approach, which is namely ARPM in this chapter, to evaluate the parameters of T and W by means of the differentiation of the energy function in equation (3) with respect to T_{pq} and W_{pq} respectively,

$$T_{pq} = \frac{\left[\sum_{i=1}^{H} \sum_{j=1}^{K} m_{ij} \left(u_{iq} - \sum_{\substack{k=1 \\ k \neq p}}^{3} v_{jk} T_{kq} - \sum_{k=1}^{K} \phi_j(v_k) W_{kq} \right) . v_{jp} \right] + \lambda_2 \delta[p-q]}{\left(\sum_{i=1}^{H} \sum_{j=1}^{K} m_{ij} v_{jp}^2 \right) + \lambda_2}$$

$$\forall 1 \leq p \leq 3, 1 \leq q \leq 3$$

$$W_{pq} = \frac{\sum_{i=1}^{H} \sum_{j=1}^{K} 2m_{ij} \left(u_{iq} - \sum_{k=1}^{3} v_{jk} T_{kq} - \sum_{\substack{k=1 \\ k \neq p}}^{K} \phi_j(v_k) W_{kq} \right) . \phi_j(v_p) - \lambda_1 \left(\sum_{\substack{k=1 \\ k \neq p}}^{K} \phi_p(v_k) W_{kq} + \sum_{\substack{k=1 \\ k \neq p}}^{K} \phi_k(v_p) W_{kq} \right)}{\left(\sum_{i=1}^{H} \sum_{j=1}^{K} 2m_{ij} \phi_j(v_p)^2 \right) + 2\lambda_1 \phi_p(v_p)}$$

$$\forall 1 \leq p \leq K, 1 \leq q \leq 3 \tag{5}$$

where $u_i = (u_{i1}, u_{i2}, u_{i3})$, $v_j = (v_{j1}, v_{j2}, v_{j3})$, $\Phi = \lfloor \phi_i(v_j) \rfloor_{K \times K}$, $T = \lfloor T_{ij} \rfloor_{3 \times 3}$, and $W = \lfloor W_{ij} \rfloor_{K \times 3}$. More specifically, W_{ij} represents the element of matrix W that is located in the pth row and in the qth column. $W = \lfloor W_{ij} \rfloor_{K \times 3}$ stands for the size of matrix W being K by 3. $\delta[n]$, the unit sample sequence, is defined: $\delta[n] = 1, \ \forall\, n = 0$; otherwise, $\delta[n] = 0, \ \forall\, n \neq 0$. The two steps are iteratively performed while the temperature parameter β as well as the weighting α is gradually decreased. The decreasing process for the temperature parameter β is similar to the deterministic annealing procedure

(Mamitsuka, 2005). The deterministic annealing with the temperature parameter β is a procedure to adjust the flexible degree of the correspondence matrix *M*. The correspondence matrix *M* eventually approaches a binary-values matrix as the temperature β is gradually annealing. In addition, due to the property that deterministic annealing can escape from the local minima, the approach is guaranteed to obtain the near-optimal solution.

2.4. Registration Refinement

After image registration, a FMLM method is proposed, which is extended from our previous work (Hsu et al., 2008), to enhance registration results to further achieve subpixel precision. The modified algorithm is better than the conventional one in efficiency because the optimization problem is reformulated so that the Hessian matrix is no longer repeatedly calculated. In addition, the proposed feature-based method is efficient since the estimate of geometric transform is from only feature points, not the whole image. It greatly reduces the computation cost and enhances the robustness of registration as well. The FMLM method converges much faster than most other methods due to its nonlinear characteristic. The sums of square intensity errors ε^2 for feature-point blocks are minimized to measure the similarity between adjacent images. It is used as the measure of convergence and is defined,

$$\begin{aligned}\varepsilon^2 &= \sum_{i=1}^{K} \sum_{x_i' \in N(x_i) \cup x_i} \left(f(x_i') - C_p(g(x_i'))\right)^2 \\ &= \sum_{fp} \left(f(x) - C_p(g(x))\right)^2,\end{aligned} \tag{6}$$

where $N(x_i)$ represents the neighborhood of the feature point x_i, K stands for the number of feature points, C_p is the geometric transform between $f(x)$ and $g(x)$ for mosaicing, and fp represents all the feature points and their neighboring points. The neighborhood of a feature point is determined according to the size of acquired image, so it is defined as a block, the size of which is between 30×30 and 40×40 in this chapter. For the adaptive geometric transform $C_p(.)$, we consider the general transform parameterized by the translation vector T_t, rotation angle R_θ, and scaling factor S_s. The geometric transform is represented by means of the operators,

$$C_p(g(x)) = C_{t,s,\theta}(g(x)) = T_t(S_s(R_\theta(g(x)))) = g(s\widetilde{\theta}\,x + t) \quad (7)$$

The sum of square errors is then derived from the FMLM algorithm,

$$\varepsilon^2 = \frac{1}{s^2}\sum\nolimits_{fp}\left(R_{-\theta}\left(S_{s^{-1}}\left(T_{-t}(f(x))\right)\right) - R_{\Delta\theta}\left(S_{1+\Delta s}\left(T_{\Delta t}(g(x))\right)\right)\right)^2, \quad (8)$$

$$\varepsilon^2 = \sum\nolimits_{fp}\left(f(x) - T_{\Delta\widetilde{\theta}(1+\Delta s)(t+\Delta t)}\left(S_{s(1+\Delta s)}\left(R_{\theta+\Delta\theta}(g(x))\right)\right)\right)^2 \quad (9)$$

where $C_{\Delta p} = (T_{\Delta t}, S_{\Delta s}, R_{\Delta\theta})$ is the update of geometric transform. The Hessian matrix A and gradient vector b are calculated,

$$\begin{aligned} b_i &= \frac{-1}{2}\frac{\partial\varepsilon^2(\Delta p)}{\partial\Delta p_i} \\ &= \frac{1}{s^2}\sum\nolimits_{fp}\left(R_{-\theta}\left(S_{s^{-1}}\left(T_{-t}(f(x))\right)\right) - R_{\Delta\theta}\left(S_{1+\Delta s}\left(T_{\Delta t}(g(x))\right)\right)\right)\frac{\partial C_{\Delta p}(g(x))}{\partial\Delta p_i} \end{aligned} \quad (10)$$

and

$$\begin{aligned} A_{ij} &= \frac{1}{2}\frac{\partial^2\varepsilon^2(\Delta p)}{\partial\Delta p_i\partial\Delta p_j} \\ &= \frac{1}{s^2}\sum\nolimits_{fp}\left(\begin{array}{l} \dfrac{\partial C_{\Delta p}(g(x))}{\partial\Delta p_i}\dfrac{\partial C_{\Delta p}(g(x))}{\partial\Delta p_j} \\ -\left(R_{-\theta}\left(S_{s^{-1}}\left(T_{-t}(f(x))\right)\right) - R_{\Delta\theta}\left(S_{1+\Delta s}\left(T_{\Delta t}(g(x))\right)\right)\right)\dfrac{\partial^2 C_{\Delta p}(g(x))}{\partial\Delta p_i\partial\Delta p_j} \end{array}\right) \end{aligned} \quad (11)$$

where $C_{\Delta p}(g(x)) = g(\Delta s\Delta\widetilde{\theta}x + \Delta t)$. As the second term in A_{ij} is small, it can be ignored.

$$\hat{A}_{ij} = \frac{1}{s^2} \sum_{fp} \frac{\partial C_{\Delta p}(g(x))}{\partial \Delta p_i} \frac{\partial C_{\Delta p}(g(x))}{\partial \Delta p_j} \tag{12}$$

Due to minimizing equation (8) with respect to Δp is the same as letting $\Delta p = 0$ in equation (9) and then minimizing it with respect to p. It is beneficial to calculate the Hessian matrix A only once as the parameter $\Delta p = 0$. Hence, the gradient vector b is rewritten as:

$$\hat{b}_i = \frac{1}{s^2} \sum_{fp} \left(R_{-\theta}\left(S_{s^{-1}}\left(T_{-t}\left(f(x)\right)\right)\right) - g(x)\right) \frac{\partial C_{\Delta p}(g(x))}{\partial \Delta p_i} \tag{13}$$

The parameter $\ddot{p}$ is then updated with estimated component Δp iteratively,

$$\ddot{p}^{(k+1)} = \ddot{p}^{(k)} + \Delta p \text{ with } \Delta p = \left(\ddot{A} + \lambda I\right)^{-1} \ddot{b}, \tag{14}$$

where λ is a positive parameter. It is adjusted according to the convergent condition of errors. The FMLM method is updated iteratively until either the relative error is below a given threshold or the number of iteration reaches a predefined value.

3. Results and Discussion

3.1. Registration Examples

The ARPM-FMLM registration algorithm is firstly applied to register several pairs of images, in which there are great differences in color difference and geometry discrepancy. These conditions, which are difficult to achieve accurate registration, are selected to test the robustness of ARPM-FMLM algorithm. They are illustrated in Figure 2. In Figure 2(a), we can observe that the slices have great inconsistency in color difference, which is usually difficult to register well with region-based registration methods. The proposed method can avoid the influence of color-difference problems and achieve successful registration. In Figure 2(b), there is a little geometry deformation in brain tissues, which would produce the noise and result in inaccurate registration.

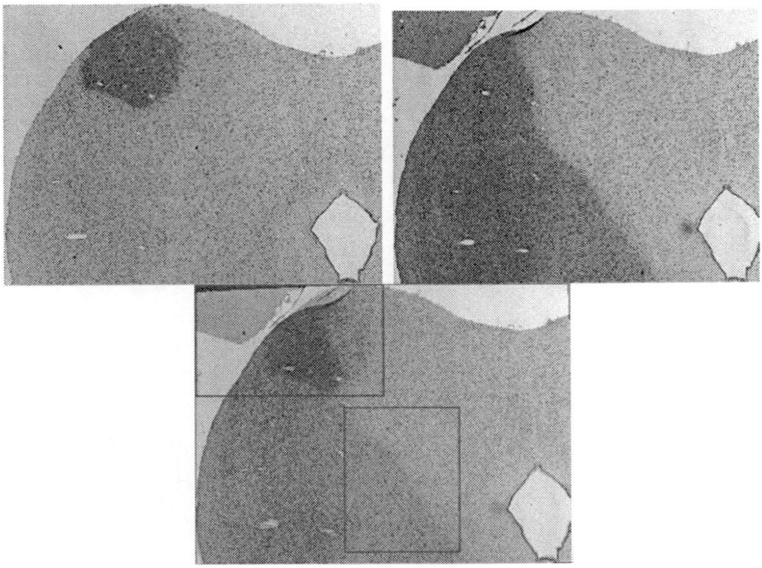

(A)

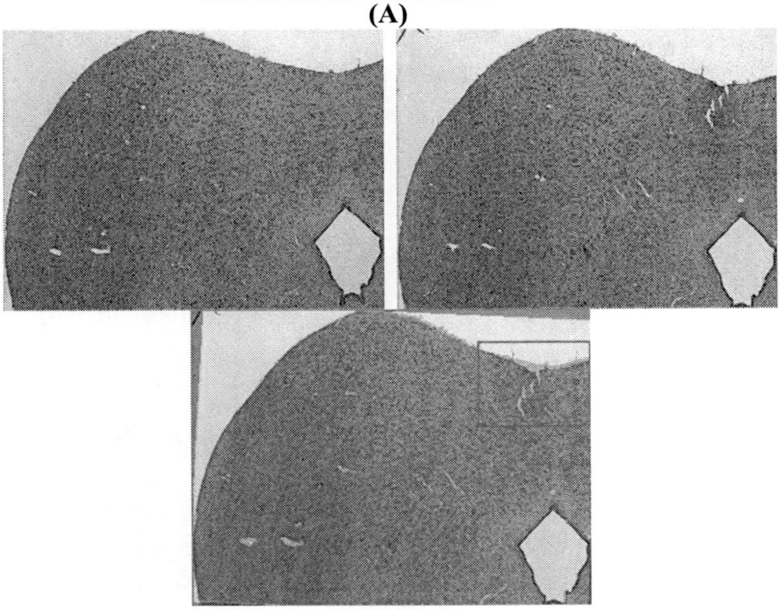

(B)

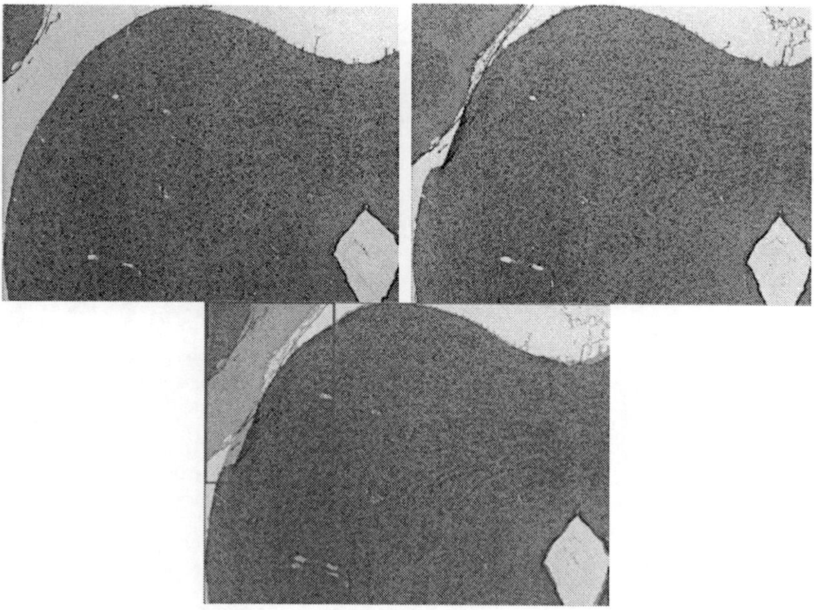

(C)

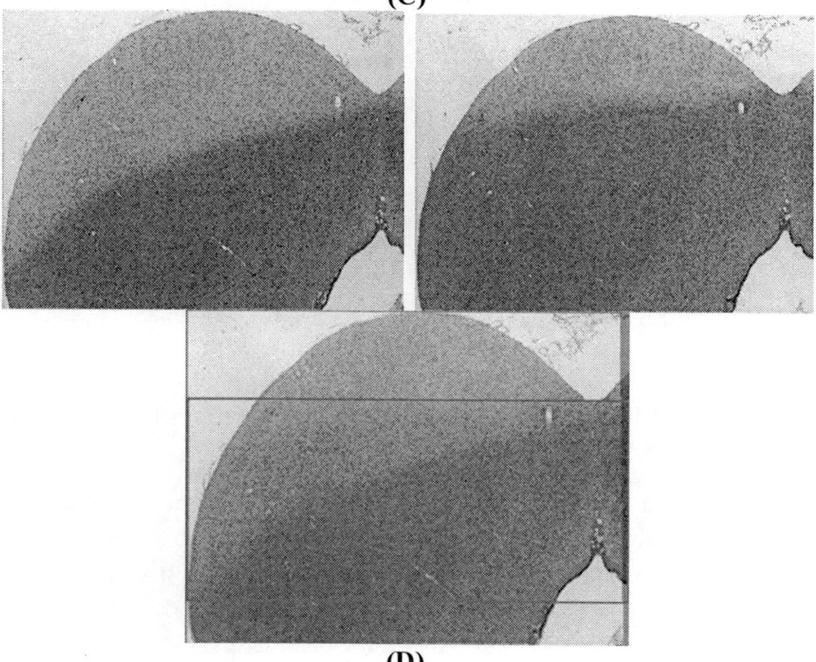

(D)

Figure 2. (Continued on next page)

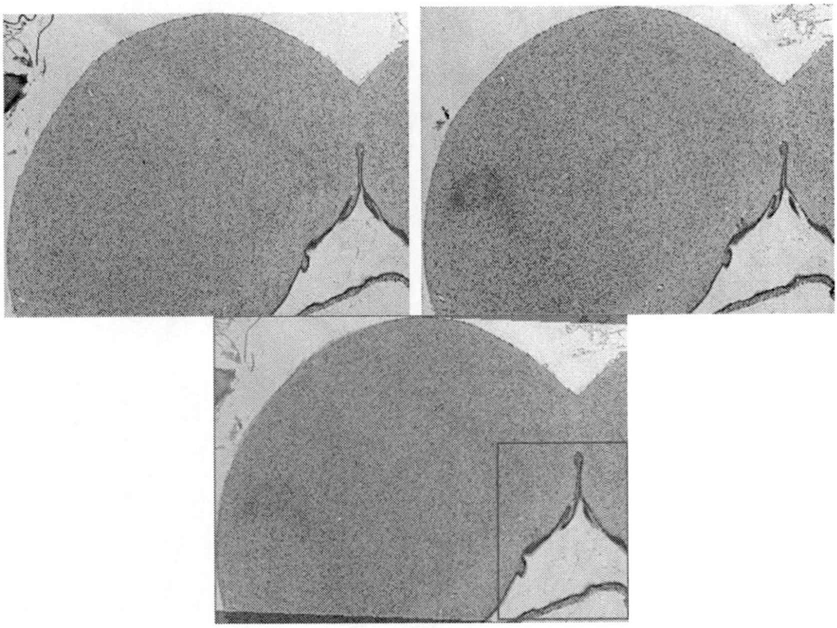

(E)

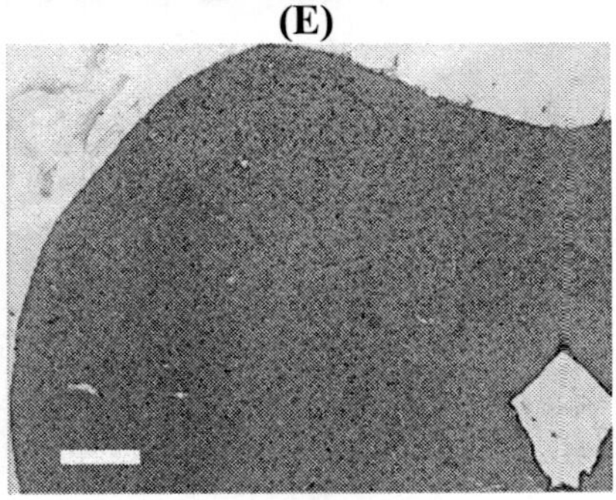

(F)

Figure 2. Registration results under the condition of great difference in color difference and geometry discrepancy; (a)-(e) registration examples; (f) scale bar (1 mm).

The proposed method can eliminate the noise as outliers and speedily achieve accurate registration by analytic evaluating the spatial correspondence and geometrical transformation. In Figure 2(c), we can see that the slices have certain geometry discrepancy, which are difficult to register accurately with general approaches. The proposed method can obtain satisfactory results due to its robustness to noise. Other registration examples are shown in Figure 2(d) and 2(e). In addition, the scale bar which represents the size of brain slices is shown in Figure 2(f). The results indicate that the ARPM-FMLM registration approach is a robust algorithm in the registration of rat brain slices.

3.2. Blood Vessel Visualization

After registration refinement, we reconstruct the volume data of rat brain from a series of microscopic images and then observe its blood vessels. A simple but effective approach, namely maximum intensity projection (MIP), is used for the vessel visualization. MIP is a volume rendering technique used to visualize high-intensity structures within volumetric data. At each pixel, the highest data value encountered along a corresponding viewing ray is depicted. MIP is commonly used to extract vascular structures from medical data sets (angiography). The results of MIP for the visualization of vessels are illustrated in Figure 3. We can observe clear shapes of slices and obvious trends of blood vessels across slices in Figure 3. MIP is a practical approach applied in view plane projection. Moreover, we can observe the trend of blood vessels by rotating reconstructed volume data along the *Z* direction. A set of projection views from volume data are shown in Figure 4.

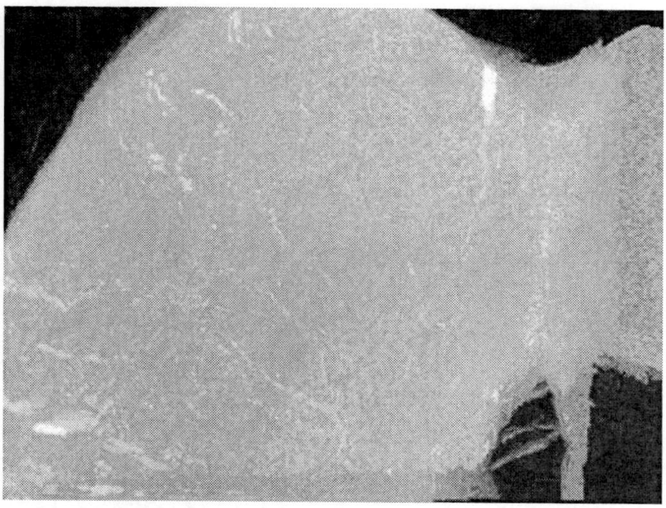

Figure 3. Blood vessel visualization.

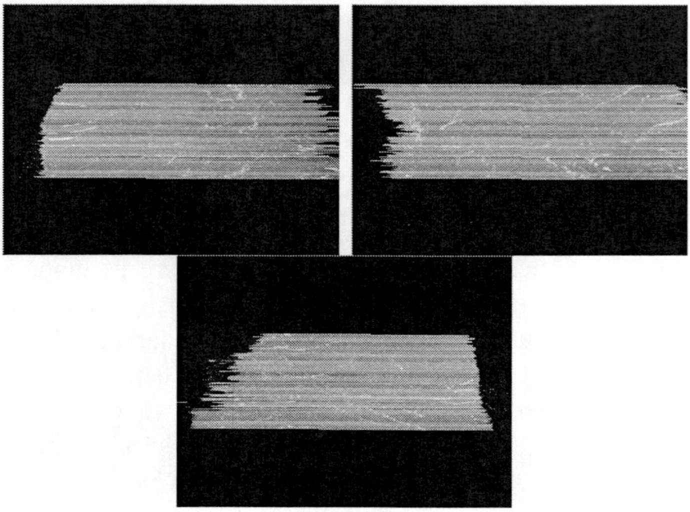

Figure 4. Blood vessel visualization by rotating reconstructed volume data along Z direction.

3.3. Quality of the Registration

We have applied the proposed registration method to all the image pairs. To assess the quality of the registration, we calculate the mean and standard deviation of the squared sum of intensity differences (*SSD*) as well as the correlation coefficient (*CC*).

$$SSD = \frac{1}{n}\sqrt{\sum (I_m - T(I_n))^2}$$

$$CC = \frac{\sum \left(I_m - \overline{I_m}\right)\left(T(I_n) - \overline{T(I_n)}\right)}{\sqrt{\sum \left(I_m - \overline{I_m}\right)^2}\sqrt{\sum \left(T(I_n) - \overline{T(I_n)}\right)^2}} \qquad (15)$$

where I_m and I_n represent a pair of images. $T(.)$ is the geometric transform evaluated after each registration step. $\overline{I_m}$ and $\overline{T(I_n)}$ denote the average intensities. n is the pixel number within the overlapping zone. For each image sequence, the *SSD* and *CC* provide an indirect measure of registration quality.

We would expect in theory that the image difference only shows the underlying noise from image acquisition. However, the effects of the misregistration, geometric deformation are clearly visible in registered images. In the experiments, we compare the proposed ARPM and ARPM-FMLM approaches with a well-known thin-plate spline robust point matching (TPS-RPM) algorithm. Figure 5 and 6 summarize the average results of registration quality in box plots in terms of *SSD* and *CC* for these three registration algorithms for synthetic and real rat brain images, respectively. Figure 5 shows the registration results for the synthetic images, which are selected from 36 rat brain images with randomly selected parameters of geometric transform, warping coefficient, and Gaussian noise. The parameters for geometric transform T are selected in the ranges of $\begin{bmatrix} N(1, 0.2) & N(0, 0.2) & N(H/10, H/30) \\ N(0, 0.2) & N(1, 0.2) & N(W/10, W/30) \\ N(0, 0.05) & N(0, 0.05) & 1 \end{bmatrix}_{3\times 3}$, where H and W represent the height and width of images, respectively; the parameters for warping coefficient W are selected in the ranges of $[N(0, 0.05)]_{K\times 3}$; the parameters for Gaussian noise are selected in the ranges of $N(0, 3 \pm 0.5)$. Figure 6 shows the registration results evaluated from 96 pairs of rat brain images. It shows that the results of the ARPM approach are similar to those of the TPS-RPM algorithm. In addition, the results also indicate that the FMLM refinement procedure can further improve the registration quality, which is better than that only the ARPM algorithm is performed.

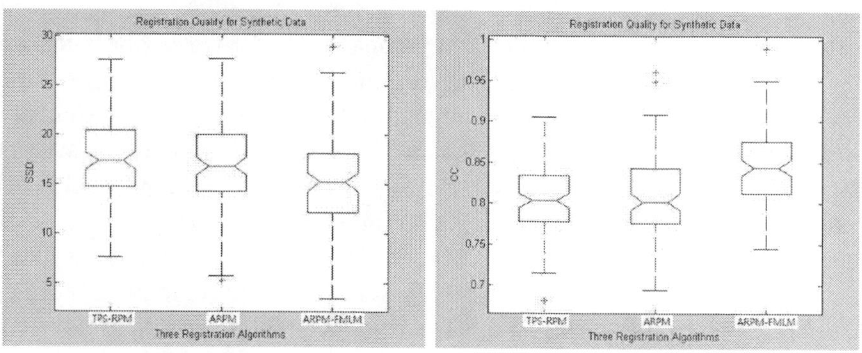

Figure 5. Comparison of average registration quality in box plots from several synthetic rat brain images in terms of SSD and CC for three registration algorithms.

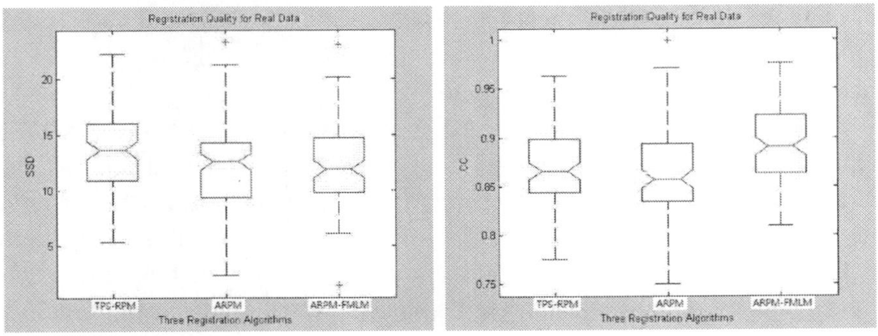

Figure 6. Comparison of average registration quality in box plots from 96 pairs of rat brain images in terms of SSD and CC for three registration algorithms.

3.4. Statistical Evaluation

To validate whether these three algorithms are significantly different or not, one-way analysis of variance (ANOVA) and multiple comparison tests are performed for the analysis of *SSD* and *CC* on both the synthetic and real data. The statistical analyses with one-way ANOVA are used to evaluate if the difference is significant for the factor *SSD* or *CC*. After analyzing with the one-way ANOVA, multiple comparison tests are used to estimate the *p*-values and significance of each pair of algorithms. We obtain *p*-values 0.0002 and less than 0.0001 for *SSD* and *CC* respectively for synthetic data, while the *p*-values are 0.013 and less than 0.0001 for *SSD* and *CC* respectively for real data. The results of test indicate that these three algorithms are significantly different among them. More detailed comparisons of *p*-values between each pair of approaches and multiple comparison tests of means are then performed. The results indicate that there are no significant differences in the estimation of *SSD* and *CC* between the ARPM and TPS-RPM algorithms for synthetic data (*p*-values be 0.5328 and 0.6441 for *SSD* and *CC*, respectively). The results also denote that the ARPM-FMLM approach is significantly better than the TPS-RPM algorithm in both *SSD* and *CC* for synthetic data (*p*-values be 0.0007 and <0.0001 for *SSD* and *CC*, respectively). In addition to synthetic data, the results of tests for real data are also discussed. The results demonstrate that there are no significant differences in *CC* estimation between the ARPM and TPS-RPM algorithms for real data, while the TPS-RPM algorithm is slightly better than the ARPM approach in *SSD* estimation (*p*-values be 0.0049 and 0.3650 for *SSD* and *CC*, respectively). The results also indicate that the ARPM-FMLM approach is better than the TPS-RPM algorithm in both *SSD* and *CC* for real data (*p*-values 0.0007 and 0.0013 for *SSD* and *CC*, respectively). Accordingly, the proposed algorithm obtains promising performance in the evaluation of registration quality for both the synthetic and real data.

3.5. Computation Time

The computation time is considered to evaluate the computational efficiency of proposed approach in this chapter. The wavelet-based feature extraction, ARPM algorithm, and FMLM refinement procedure take approximately one, nine, and six minutes to complete the registration of a microscopic image sequence on an Intel Core 2 Duo E6300 computer system, respectively. More specifically, the amount of data that the proposed approach is able to process per time unit is about 74.6 images and corresponding 16218.0 feature points per minute for wavelet-based feature extraction, 10.8 image pairs and corresponding 1774.4 feature-point pairs per minute for ARPM algorithm, and 15.7 image pairs and corresponding 2579.5 feature-point pairs per minute for FMLM refinement procedure. It indicates that the proposed method is less time consuming in computation cost.

CONCLUSION

In this chapter, we have presented a robust registration algorithm for the reconstruction of rat brain. The concept that features could exist in multiscale is applied to determine which true feature points are. The ARPM algorithm combined with the FMLM refinement procedure are proposed to speedily achieve registration accuracy and robust to the influence of color difference and geometry discrepancy at the same time. Several pairs of images of great differences in color difference and geometry discrepancy are selected for the test, and the proposed method obtains good results. In the evaluation of registration quality in terms of *SSD* and *CC*, the proposed method also achieves promising performance for both the synthetic and real data. In addition, the proposed method is less time consuming in computation cost. It shows that this chapter is really valuable for equipping the biologists and doctors with a powerful tool in registration applications. In future work, we will address the issue of registration in different modal and multi-modality images.

ACKNOWLEDGMENTS

The author would like to express his appreciation for shared facilities supported by the Program of Top 100 Universities Advancement, Ministry of Education, Taiwan.

REFERENCES

Chakravarty MM, Bertrand G, Hodge CP, Sadikot AF, Collins DL. 2006. The creation of a brain atlas for image guided neurosurgery using serial histological data. *Neuroimage* 30:359-376.

Chetverikov D, Stepanov D, Krsek P. 2005. Robust Euclidean alignment of 3D point sets: the trimmed iterative closest point algorithm. *Image and Vision Computing* 23:299-309.

Chui H, Rangarajan A. 2003. A new point matching algorithm for non-rigid registration. *Computer Vision and Image Understanding* 89:114–141.

Cornillie P, Van Den Broeck W, Simoens P. 2008. Three-dimensional reconstruction of the remodeling of the systemic vasculature in early pig embryos. *Microsc Res Tech* 71:105–111.

DâââAgostino E, Maes F, Vandermeulen D, Suetens P. 2006. An information theoretic approach for non-rigid image registration using voxel class probabilities. *Medical Image Analysis* 10:413-431.

Droske M, Rumpf M. 2007. Multiscale Joint Segmentation and Registration of Image Morphology. *IEEE Trans. Pattern Anal. Machine Intell.* 29:2181-2194.

Fernandez-Gonzalez R, Jones A, Garcia-Rodriguez E, Chen PY, Idica A, Lockett SJ, Barcellos-Hoff MH, Ortiz-De-Solorzano C. 2002. System for combined three-dimensional morphological and molecular analysis of thick tissue specimens. *Microsc Res Tech* 59:522–530.

Foroughi P, Abolmaesumi P, Hashtrudi-Zaad K. 2006. Intra-subject elastic registration of 3D ultrasound images. *Medical Image Analysis* 10:713-725.

Gefen S, Kiryati N, Nissanov J. 2008. Atlas-based indexing of brain sections via 2-d to 3-d image registration. *IEEE Trans. Biomedical Engineering* 55:147-156.

Gholipour A, Kehtarnavaz N, Briggs R, Devous M, Gopinath K. 2007. Brain functional localization: A survey of image registration techniques. *IEEE Trans. Med. Imag.* 26:427-451.

Han X, Xu C, Prince JL. 2003. A topology preserving level set method for geometric deformable models. *IEEE Trans. Pattern Anal. Machine Intell.* 25:755–768.

Holden M. 2008. A review of geometric transformations for nonrigid body registration. *IEEE Trans. Med. Imag.* 27:111–128.

Hsieh JW, Liao HYM, Fan KC, Ko MT, Hung YP. 1997. Image registration using a new edge-based approach. *Computer Vision and Image Understanding* 67:112–130.

Hsu WY, Poon WFP, Sun YN. 2008. Automatic seamless mosaicing of microscopic images: Enhancing appearance with color degradation compensation and wavelet-based blending. *Journal of Microscopy* 231:408-418.

Klein S, Staring M, Murphy K, Viergever MA, Pluim J. 2010. Elastix: A toolbox for intensity-based medical image registration. *IEEE Trans. Med. Imag.* 29:196–205.

Lebenberg J, Hérard AS, Dubois A, Dauguet J, Frouin V, Dhenain M, Hantraye P, Delzescaux T. 2010. Validation of MRI-based 3D digital atlas registration with histological and autoradiographic volumes: an anatomofunctional transgenic mouse brain imaging study. *Neuroimage.* 51:1037-1046.

Loeckx D, Slagmolen P, Maes F, Vandermeulen D, Suetens P. 2010. Nonrigid image registration using conditional mutual information. *IEEE Trans. Med. Imag.* 29:19-29.

Mamitsuka H. 2005. Finding the biologically optimal alignment of multiple sequences. *Artificial intelligence in medicine* 35:9-18.

Shu L, Chung ACS. 2010. Feature based nonrigid brain MR image registration with symmetric alpha stable filters. *IEEE Trans. Med. Imag.* 29:106-119.

Simonetti AW, Elezi VA, Farion R, Malandain G, Segebartha C, Remy C, Barbier EL. 2006. A low temperature embedding and section registration strategy for 3D image reconstruction of the rat brain from autoradiographic sections. *Journal of Neuroscience Methods* 158:242–250.

Walimbe V, Shekhar R. 2006. Automatic elastic image registration by interpolation of 3D rotations and translations from discrete rigid-body transformations. *Medical Image Analysis* 10:899-914.

Yelnik J, Bardinet E, Dormont D, Malandain G, Ourselin S, Tandé D, Karachi C, Ayache N, Cornu P, Agid Y. 2007. A three-dimensional, histological and deformable atlas of the human basal ganglia. I. Atlas construction based on immunohistochemical and MRI data. *Neuroimage* 34:618-638.

Zacharaki EI, Hogea CS, Biros G, Davatzikos C. 2008. A comparative study of biomechanical simulators in deformable registration of brain tumor images. *IEEE Trans. Biomedical Engineering* 55:1233-1236.

Zheng Y, Doermann D. 2006. Robust point matching for nonrigid shapes by preserving local neighborhood structures. *IEEE Trans. Pattern Anal. Machine Intell.* 28:643-649.

In: Medical Imaging
Editors: M. D'Elia and A. Madaffari
ISBN: 978-1-62081-049-1

Chapter 3

UTILITY OF WHOLE-BODY FLUORINE-18-FLUORODEOXYGLUCOSE POSITRON EMISSION TOMOGRAPHY IN PATIENTS WITH SARCOIDOSIS

Giorgio Treglia*, Silvia Taralli,
Maria Vittoria Mattoli and Alessandro Giordano
Institute of Nuclear Medicine, Department of Bioimaging and Radiological Sciences, Catholic University of the Sacred Heart, Rome, Italy

ABSTRACT

Objective: to review the emerging role of whole-body positron emission tomography (PET) and positron emission tomography / computed tomography (PET/CT) with Fluorine-18-Fluorodeoxyglucose (FDG) in patients with sarcoidosis.

Methods: A literature search of published studies regarding whole-body FDG-PET and PET/CT in patients with sarcoidosis was performed.

Results: Main findings of the scientific literature are reported and discussed.

* Corresponding Author and reprint requests: Dr. Giorgio Treglia, Institute of Nuclear Medicine, Positron Emission Tomography Centre, Department of Bioimaging and Radiological Sciences, Catholic University of the Sacred Heart. Address: Largo Gemelli, 8; Rome, Italy. Zip code: 00168. Email address: giorgiomednuc@libero.it. fax number: 0039063013745. telephone: 00390630154978.

Conclusions: Positive FDG-PET findings should be interpreted with caution in differentiating sarcoidosis from other inflammatory diseases and malignant abnormalities. FDG-PET seems to be a very useful molecular imaging method in assessing disease activity, in staging and identifying occult sites, and in monitoring treatment response in patients with sarcoidosis. FDG-PET shows a better diagnostic accuracy compared to Gallium-67 scintigraphy in patients with sarcoidosis, in addition to several practical advantages.

Keywords: Positron emission tomography, ^{18}F-FDG, sarcoidosis.

INTRODUCTION

Imaging methods may play a role in diagnosis and treatment strategy plan in patients with sarcoidosis at both primary staging and follow-up. Chest radiography and computed tomography (CT) may support the diagnosis of sarcoidosis. Bilateral pulmonary hilar and mediastinal lymphadenopathy is the most common radiological finding, often associated with pulmonary infiltrates [1-5]. About functional imaging methods, Gallium-67 (^{67}Ga) scintigraphy is not routinely used in patients with sarcoidosis. This method has several limitations: a) it is a time consuming method (patients must be injected at least 48-72 hours before image acquisition); b) there is a significant interobserver variability in image interpretation; c) the overall sensitivity and specificity values are highly variable between different studies; d) this scintigraphic method yields a high radiation exposure [3,6,7].

While whole-body ^{18}F-fluorodeoxyglucose positron emission tomography (FDG-PET) is reported to be a sensitive technique in oncological imaging, it is well known that inflammatory and infectious lesions may cause false positive results [8,9]. Inflammatory cells such as macrophages, lymphocytes and neutrophil granulocytes as well as fibroblasts have shown to avidly take up FDG. Therefore, FDG may also be used as a tracer of inflammation [6,7,10,11].

FDG enters the cell by the same membrane transport mechanism as glucose. After penetration of the cellular membrane via glucose transporters, both FDG and glucose are phosphorylated by an hexokinase. Unlike glucose-6-phosphate, FDG-6-phosphate is not a substrate of glucose-6-phosphate isomerase and does not undergo further metabolism in the glucose pathway; FDG is therefore trapped within cells.

Autoradiographic studies of FDG uptake in sarcoidosis are lacking and the specific cell type(s) remain unknown, although it is well known that FDG is incorporated in inflammatory cells.

Disease activity in sarcoidosis can be assessed by detecting and quantifying the degree of inflammatory and granulomatous reactions that occur in the lungs and elsewhere in the body. The ability to visualize FDG accumulation by activated inflammatory cells makes whole-body FDG-PET a promising modality for assess disease activity in patients with sarcoidosis, as first described by the report of Lewis and Salama in 1994 [12].

Several studies have shown the potential role of whole-body FDG-PET in evaluating disease activity in patients with sarcoidosis. A literature search of published studies regarding whole-body FDG-PET and PET/CT in patients with sarcoidosis was performed.

METHODS

A comprehensive computer literature search was conducted to find relevant published articles about whole-body FDG-PET in patients with sarcoidosis; the search was updated until April 2011. Main findings of the literature were reported and discussed.

RESULTS

A) Literature Data

In 1998 *Yamada et al* [13] evaluated the role of different PET tracers, FDG and ^{11}C-Methionine (Met), an amino acid tracer, in clinical assessment of thoracic lymph nodal involvement in 31 patients with pulmonary sarcoidosis. Clinical reassessment of sarcoidosis was made at least one year after the first PET examination. Overall sensitivities of FDG and Met-PET in detecting thoracic lymphadenopathy were both 97% (30/31 patients). The mean FDG uptake value was significantly higher than mean Met uptake value ($p<0.01$). Dividing the patients into two groups, the FDG-dominant group (FDG/Met uptake ratio ≥ 2), and the Met-dominant group (FDG/Met uptake ratio < 2) there was a significant linear correlation between FDG and Met uptake values in each group (FDG-dominant group, $r=0.93$, $p<0.01$; Met-dominant group,

$r=0.41$, $p<0.01$). Patients did not receive any treatment after the PET scan. The FDG-dominant group showed a significantly greater remission incidence of thoracic lymphadenopathy compared to the Met-dominant group (78% versus 33%; $p<0.05$). The incidence of unchanged lymphadenopathy plus that of the appearance of pulmonary involvement, assessed by CT, was higher in the Met- (67%) than in the FDG-dominant group (22%). These findings suggest that: 1) both FDG and Met are accumulated in mediastinal and hilar lymph nodes in patients with sarcoidosis, suggesting that sarcoid lymph nodes have a high metabolic demand for both glucose and amino acids; 2) the different uptake of FDG and Met in thoracic lymph nodes would provide information about short term prognosis for sarcoidosis patients: the disease activity seems to decrease over time without treatment giving a good prognosis for the FDG-dominant group; on the other hand, the disease activity is likely to continue, resulting in pulmonary involvement, and giving a poor prognosis for the Met-dominant group.

In 2006 *Nishiyama et al* [14] compared FDG-PET and ^{67}Ga scintigraphy in the evaluation of pulmonary and extrapulmonary involvement in patients with sarcoidosis. Eighteen patients with sarcoidosis were examined; FDG and ^{67}Ga uptake were visually and semiquantitatively evaluated. The presence of pulmonary and extrapulmonary lesions was evaluated by histopathology or radiological findings. Five patients had only pulmonary lesions, 12 patients had both pulmonary and extrapulmonary lesions, and one patient had only extrapulmonary lesions. Both planar and tomographic (SPECT) ^{67}Ga images detected 17 of 21 (81%) clinically observed pulmonary sites. Planar ^{67}Ga images detected 15 of 31 (48%) clinically observed extrapulmonary sites. FDG-PET detected all 21 (100%) clinically observed pulmonary sites and 28 of 31 (90%) clinically observed extrapulmonary sites. When correlated with clinical and radiological follow-up, FDG or ^{67}Ga uptake in pulmonary and extrapulmonary lesions was decreased after corticosteroid therapy. These results suggest that FDG-PET can detect pulmonary lesions to a similar degree as ^{67}Ga scintigraphy in patients with sarcoidosis. However, FDG-PET appears to be more accurate and contributes to a better evaluation of extrapulmonary involvement in patients with sarcoidosis. FDG-PET appears to be preferable in patients with sarcoidosis, compared to ^{67}Ga scintigraphy, because of at least comparable and perhaps even better sensitivity of FDG-PET in addition to several practical advantages (less radiation exposure, shorter time between injection and imaging).

In 2007 *Kaira et al* [15] investigated the usefulness of PET with ^{18}F-methyltyrosine (FMT), an amino acid tracer used for detecting neoplasms, in combination with FDG-PET for the diagnosis of sarcoidosis in patients with suspected malignancy. Twenty-four sarcoidosis patients with suspected malignancy underwent FDG and FMT-PET. The study included 17 patients with extrapulmonary lesions mimicking malignant disease, three patients with occurrence of bilateral hilar lymphadenopathy, and four patients with multiple nodules mimicking pulmonary metastasis. All patients showed increased FDG uptake and no increased FMT uptake in their lymphadenopathies. All extranodal lesions such as liver, spleen, and bone were visually positive on FDG-PET and negative on FMT-PET. No neoplasm was confirmed in all patients. These results suggest that FDG-PET is positive in sarcoid lesions, and therefore this method could not differentiate sarcoidosis from malignant disease. Use of FMT-PET in combination with FDG-PET may be the effective method to distinguish sarcoidosis from malignancy.

In 2007 *Teirstein et al* [16] studied the role FDG-PET in the identification of occult sites and reversible granulomatous disease in patients with sarcoidosis. A total of 188 FDG-PET scans performed in 137 patients with proven sarcoidosis were retrospectively reviewed. A total of 139 of 188 FDG-PET scans (74%) were positive. The most common positive sites were mediastinal lymph nodes (54 scans), extrathoracic lymph nodes (30 scans), and lung (24 scans). Twenty occult disease sites were identified. A total of 36 patients were treated, but only 11 patients exhibited decreased FDG uptake with corticosteroid therapy. The positive pulmonary FDG-PET scan findings occurred in two-thirds of patients with radiographic stage II and III sarcoidosis. Negative pulmonary FDG-PET scan findings were common in patients with radiographic stage 0, I, and IV. These findings suggest that FDG-PET is a valuable tool in identifying occult sites in patients with sarcoidosis and in assessing residual activity in patients with fibrotic pulmonary sarcoidosis.

In 2008 *Prager et al* [17] analyzed possible advantages of FDG-PET over ^{67}Ga scintigraphy during the primary assessment of patients with sarcoidosis. Twenty-four patients with histologically proven sarcoidosis were investigated with both methods. There was a significant difference in the detection of pulmonary and extrapulmonary sarcoidosis lesions between planar ^{67}Ga scintigraphy and FDG-PET images ($p<0.002$): a total of 64 lesions were detected with ^{67}Ga scintigraphy in the thorax and elsewhere, while 85 lesions were found with FDG-PET. There was complete agreement between FDG-PET and ^{67}Ga scintigraphy in thoracic manifestations in four (16.6%) patients, and in non-thoracic manifestations in five (20.8%) patients. In 10/24 (41.6%) patients, FDG-PET revealed more affected foci in thoracic sarcoidosis than

^{67}Ga scintigraphy, in non-thoracic disease in 7/24 (29.1%) patients. In conclusion ^{67}Ga and FDG are useful tracers for diagnostic evaluation of thoracic sarcoidosis, but FDG seems to be more suitable for imaging the mediastinum, the bi-hilar lymph nodes, the posterior regions of the lungs and non-thoracic lesions.

In 2008 *Braun et al* [18] evaluated the role of FDG-PET/CT for diagnosis and therapeutic follow-up of patients with sarcoidosis. Twenty patients with biopsy-proven sarcoidosis were retrospectively included, in particular, 13 and seven cases of thoracic and extra-thoracic sarcoidosis, respectively. All patients underwent FDG-PET/CT, and 12 of them also ^{67}Ga scintigraphy. Both FDG-PET/CT and ^{67}Ga scintigraphy highlighted multiple extra-thoracic foci of pathological tracer uptake, suggesting the presence of active granulomatous disease, which was not previously detected by conventional evaluation. Considering both thoracic and extra-thoracic sarcoidosis localizations, FDG-PET/CT sensitivity was 78% (28 out of 36 biopsy-proven sites of sarcoidosis were correctly identified). For thoracic, sinonasal, and pharyngolaryngeal localizations, FDG-PET/CT sensitivity was 100%, 100%, and 80%, respectively. Considering only the 12 patients who underwent both scintigraphic examinations, overall sensitivity of ^{67}Ga scintigraphy and FDG-PET/CT was 58% and 79%, respectively and improved to 67% and 86% after excluding all sites of skin involvement. To evaluate the efficacy of corticosteroid treatment, five enrolled patients underwent a second FDG-PET/CT. Complete regression of all foci of pathological tracer uptake was showed in two cases, allowing therapy withdrawal; improvement but incomplete regression of mediastinal-pulmonary disease occurred in two patients; disease progression was assessed in one patient. These results suggest that FDG-PET/CT allows to obtain a complete morpho-functional map of inflammatory active localizations and to follow treatment efficacy in patients with sarcoidosis, particularly in atypical, complex, and systemic forms. The better quality of imaging, the less technical constraints and better sensitivity are in favor of FDG-PET/CT compared to ^{67}Ga scintigraphy in this field.

In 2008 *Keijsers et al* [19] correlated FDG-PET with standard sarcoidosis activity parameters during infliximab treatment (anti-TNF-α therapy) in order to illustrate that FDG uptake represents active disease and might be used to monitor therapeutic effects. Twelve patients with refractory sarcoidosis were treated with 6 cycles of infliximab. Pre- and post-therapy FDG-PET was visually and semiquantitative evaluated: standardized uptake value (SUVmax) was measured. In addition, the effect of infliximab was evaluated by changes in symptoms, angiotensin converting enzyme (ACE), soluble interleukin-2 receptor (sIL-2R), vital capacity (VC), diffusion capacity of the lung for carbon monoxide (DLCO) and chest radiography. SUVmax and conventional parameters were correlated. Clinical improvement as judged by conventional parameters was seen in all patients, though with a minor response in one. Symptoms improved in 11/12 patients while chest radiographic stages did not change. Pre-infliximab FDG-PET was abnormal in all patients: involvement of the pulmonary tract was seen in all 12 patients, while eight patients showed extrapulmonary involvement. Post-infliximab FDG-PET revealed either improvement or normalization in 11/12 (92%) clinically responding patients. The overall decrease in SUVmax was 55% ($p<0.01$); the patient with a limited response showed a 34% increase of SUVmax. A decrease in SUVmax of the lung parenchyma correlated with an improvement of VC ($r=-0.75$, $p<0.01$). No significant correlation between SUVmax and other parameters was found. These results suggest that changes imaged by FDG-PET during infliximab treatment in patients with sarcoidosis correlate with signs of clinical improvement, which supports the hypothesis that FDG uptake represents disease activity and may be used to monitor therapeutic effects.

In 2009 *Keijsers et al* [20] determined the sensitivity of FDG-PET in active sarcoidosis and its correlation with serological markers widely used for determining sarcoidosis activity, angiotensin-converting enzyme (ACE) and soluble interleukin-2 receptor (sIL-2R). This retrospective study included 36 newly diagnosed, symptomatic sarcoidosis patients. FDG-PET was visually and semiquantitatively evaluated: maximum and average standardized uptake values (SUVmax and SUVavg) were compared with ACE and sIL-2R. FDG-PET was found positive in 34 of 36 patients (94%). Of the 32 patients with pulmonary involvement, extrapulmonary lesions were seen in 19 patients. Two patients had extrapulmonary lesions without pulmonary involvement. Thus, a total of 21 patients (58%) had extrapulmonary involvement. Thirteen patients (36%) showed an increased ACE value; seventeen patients (47%) showed an increased sIL-2R value. No correlation was found between SUV and ACE or sIL-2R values. Of the 34 patients with a positive FDG-PET result, 12 patients showed an increased ACE value (35%) and 16 patients showed an increased sIL-2R value (47%). Fourteen patients had a negative ACE as well as sIL-2R value (41%). Of 13 patients with an increased ACE value, 12 showed a positive FDG-PET (92%); of 17 patients with an increased sIL-2R value, 16 showed a positive FDG-PET (94%). These findings demonstrated that-FDG-PET is a very sensitive technique to assess disease activity in sarcoidosis, in contrast with ACE and sIL-2R values, suggesting a pivotal role for FDG-PET in sarcoidosis assessment. Positive ACE and sIL-2R correlate well with FDG-

PET, suggesting that FDG-PET might be omitted when these serum markers are elevated.

In 2010 *Keijsers et al* [21] compared FDG-PET with bronchoalveolar lavage (BAL) cell profiles patterns to assess whether metabolic activity imaged by FDG-PET represents disease activity as reflected by BAL. A total of 77 newly diagnosed pulmonary sarcoidosis patients underwent BAL and FDG-PET. Based on FDG-PET, patients were diagnosed with exclusively mediastinal/hilar activity (group A) and activity in the lung parenchyma (group B). Per group, BAL lymphocytes (%), CD4/CD8 ratio, $CD103^{+}CD4^{+}/CD4^{+}$ ratio and neutrophils (%) were compared with the extent of metabolic activity expressed as the maximum standardized uptake value (SUVmax). Additionally, SUVmax and BAL parameters per radiographic stage were analysed. FDG-PET was positive in 75 patients (97%) and 73 of them demonstrated thoracic involvement (95%). Mediastinal/hilar activity was present in all 73 patients, which was accompanied by parenchymal activity in 50 patients. There were no patients with increased activity in the lung parenchyma without mediastinal/hilar involvement. Group A (exclusively mediastinal/hilar activity) consisted of 23 patients. Group B (increased metabolic activity in the lung parenchyma) consisted of 50 patients. Overall, SUVmax in the lung parenchyma significantly correlated with the percentage of neutrophils ($r=0.38$, $p<0.01$); SUVmax of the mediastinum/hila significantly correlated with the CD4/CD8 ratio ($r=0.39$, $p<0.01$); a negative correlation between the SUVmax of the mediastinum/hila and the $CD103^{+}CD4^{+}/CD4^{+}$ ratio ($r=-0.39$, $p<0.01$) was found. The SUVmax of the lung parenchyma was positively related to the radiographic stage, while the SUVmax of the mediastinum/hila and CD4/CD8 ratio were inversely related. These results suggest that FDG-PET correlates with the CD4/CD8 ratio and neutrophils, suggesting that FDG-PET represents this specific cell profile in BAL. High SUVmax values of the lung parenchyma may correlate with more severe parenchymal involvement, particularly when accompanied by a low SUVmax of the mediastinum/hila.

Recently, *Keijsers et al* [22] investigated the sensitivity of ^{67}Ga imaging and FDG-PET for sarcoidosis activity and their interobserver variability. Thirty-four newly diagnosed, histologically proven sarcoidosis patients were analyzed prospectively. Overall sensitivity to detect active sarcoidosis was 88% for ^{67}Ga imaging and 97% for FDG-PET. Although these results were not significantly different, FDG-PET detected more lesions in the mediastinum ($p<0.05$), hila ($p<0.05$), lymph nodes ($p<0.001$) and extrapulmonary regions in general ($p<0.001$). Interobserver agreement was poor to moderate for ^{67}Ga imaging (kappa 0.19-0.59) and good to very good for FDG-PET (kappa 0.65-1.00). These findings demonstrate that FDG-PET should be considered the nuclear imaging technique of choice in sarcoidosis assessment.

B) Problems and Limitations

Literature findings support current concepts which are integrated in clinical practice and management in patients with sarcoidosis.Sarcoidosis has an interesting geographic distribution relative to other diseases such as tuberculosis, fungal infections as well as clinical and radiologic presentation patterns. These characteristics decrease specificity of FDG-PET for sarcoidosis and makes interpretation of PET images difficult.

Furthermore FDG-PET cannot distinguish between inflammatory and malignant lesions, both usually characterized by increased FDG uptake. For these reasons FDG-PET is best used to monitor the disease in patients with proven sarcoidosis, while diagnosis always requires histologic confirmation.

It should be considered that FDG-PET is an imaging method characterized by relatively higher costs and lower availability compared to other imaging methods such as CT.In this review only whole-body PET studies in patients with sarcoidosis were included; studies about the role of FDG-PET in patients with cardiac sarcoidosis were not included. Currently, there are not validated studies of FDG-PET in cardiac sarcoidosis; the main problem is the physiologic uptake of FDG in myocardium, perhaps solved by a carbohydrate restricted diet.Another problem is the lack of sufficient studies that evaluated the role of FDG-PET in detecting sarcoidosis in certain organs (for example skin, liver, gastrointestinal tract, nervous system), potential sites of missed sarcoidosis lesions with FDG-PET.A possible limitation of this review is the small number of studies and the small number of patients included in each study which may influence the conclusions. Also, to date, Medicare decided to not reimburse FDG-PET for the assessment of sarcoidosis, based on insufficient data. Further studies with a larger patient population are needed to correctly define the role of FDG-PET in patients with sarcoidosis.

Conclusion

From this review of the literature about the role of FDG-PET in patients with sarcoidosis we conclude that:

1) Positive FDG-PET findings should be interpreted with caution in differentiating sarcoidosis from other inflammatory diseases and malignant abnormalities;
2) FDG-PET seems to be a very useful molecular imaging method in assessing disease activity, in staging and identifying occult sites, and in monitoring treatment response in patients with sarcoidosis;
3) FDG-PET shows a better diagnostic accuracy compared to ^{67}Ga scintigraphy in patients with sarcoidosis, because of a better sensitivity of FDG-PET (mainly due to the high quality of FDG-PET images with superior contrast and spatial resolution compared to ^{67}Ga scintigraphy) in addition to several practical advantages (less radiation exposure, shorter time between injection and imaging).

REFERENCES

[1] Morgenthau AS, Iannuzzi MC. Recent advances in sarcoidosis. *Chest*, 2011;139:174-182.

[2] Iannuzzi MC, Rybicki BA, Teirstein AS. Sarcoidosis. *N. Engl. J. Med.*,. 2007;357:2153-2165.

[3] ATS/ERS/WASOG Committee. Statement on Sarcoidosis. *Sarcoidosis Vasc. Diffuse Lung Dis.*, 1999;16:149-173.

[4] Nunes H, Soler P, Valeyre D. Pulmonary sarcoidosis. *Allergy*, 2005;60:565-582.

[5] Koyama T, Ueda H, Togashi K, Umeoka S, Kataoka M, Nagai S. Radiologic manifestations of sarcoidosis in various organs. *Radiographics*, 2004;24:87-104.

[6] Gotthardt M, Bleeker-Rovers CP, Boerman OC, Oyen WJ. Imaging of inflammation by PET, conventional scintigraphy, and other imaging techniques. *J. Nucl. Med.,* 2010;51:1937-1949.

[7] Basu S, Zhuang H, Torigian DA, Rosenbaum J, Chen W, Alavi A. Functional imaging of inflammatory diseases using nuclear medicine techniques. *Semin. Nucl. Med.*, 2009;39:124-145.

[8] Bakheet S, Powe J. Benign causes of 18-FDG uptake on whole-body imaging. *Semin. Nucl. Med.*, 2000;28:352-358.

[9] Kubota R, Yamada S, Kubota K, Ishiwata K, Tamahashi N, Ido T. Intratumoral distribution of fluorine-18-deoxyglucose in vivo: high accumulation in macrophages and granulation tissues studied by microautoradiography. *J. Nucl. Med.*, 1992;33:1972-1980.

[10] Bleeker-Rovers CP, Vos FJ, Corstens FH, Oyen WJ. Imaging of infectious diseases using [18F] fluorodeoxyglucose PET. *Q. J. Nucl. Med. Mol. Imaging.* 2008;52:17-29.

[11] Treglia G, Cason E, Fagioli G. Recent applications of nuclear medicine in diagnostics: II part. *Italian Journal of Medicine,* 2010;4:159-166.

[12] Lewis PJ, Salama A. Uptake of fluorine-18-fluorodeoxyglucose in sarcoidosis. *J. Nucl. Med.,* 1994;35:1647-1649.

[13] Yamada Y, Uchida Y, Tatsumi K, Yamaguchi T, Kimura H, Kitahara H, Kuriyama T. Fluorine-18-fluorodeoxyglucose and carbon-11-methionine evaluation of lymphadenopathy in sarcoidosis. *J. Nucl. Med.,* 1998;39:1160-1166.

[14] Nishiyama Y, Yamamoto Y, Fukunaga K, Takinami H, Iwado Y, Satoh K, Ohkawa M. Comparative evaluation of 18F-FDG-PET and 67Ga scintigraphy in patients with sarcoidosis. *J. Nucl. Med.,* 2006;47:1571-1576.

[15] Kaira K, Oriuchi N, Otani Y, Yanagitani N, Sunaga N, Hisada T, Ishizuka T, Endo K, Mori M. Diagnostic usefulness of fluorine-18-alpha-methyltyrosine positron emission tomography in combination with 18F-fluorodeoxyglucose in sarcoidosis patients. *Chest,* 2007;131:1019-1027.

[16] Teirstein AS, Machac J, Almeida O, Lu P, Padilla ML, Iannuzzi MC. Results of 188 whole-body fluorodeoxyglucose positron emission tomography scans in 137 patients with sarcoidosis. *Chest,* 2007;132:1949-1953.

[17] Prager E, Wehrschuetz M, Bisail B, Woltsche M, Schwarz T, Lanz H, Sorantin E, Aigner RM. Comparison of 18F-FDG and 67Ga-citrate in sarcoidosis imaging. *Nuklearmedizin,* 2008;47:18-23.

[18] Braun JJ, Kessler R, Constantinesco A, Imperiale A. 18F-FDG-PET/CT in sarcoidosis management: review and report of 20 cases. *Eur. J. Nucl. Med. Mol. Imaging.,* 2008;35:1537-1543.

[19] Keijsers RG, Verzijlbergen JF, van Diepen DM, van den Bosch JM, Grutters JC. 18F-FDG-PET in sarcoidosis: an observational study in 12 patients treated with infliximab. *Sarcoidosis Vasc. Diffuse Lung Dis.,* 2008;25:143-149.

[20] Keijsers RG, Verzijlbergen FJ, Oyen WJ, van den Bosch JM, Ruven HJ, vanVelzen-Blad H, Grutters JC. 18F-FDG-PET, genotype-corrected ACE and sIL-2R in newly diagnosed sarcoidosis. *Eur. J. Nucl. Med. Mol. Imaging.,* 2009;36:1131-1137.

[21] Keijsers RG, Grutters JC, van Velzen-Blad H, van den Bosch JM, Oyen WJ, Verzijlbergen FJ. (18)F-FDG-PET patterns and BAL cell profiles in pulmonary sarcoidosis. *Eur. J. Nucl. Med. Mol. Imaging.,* 2010;37:1181-1188.

[22] Keijsers RG, Grutters JC, Thomeer M, Du Bois RM, Van Buul MM, Lavalaye J, Van Den Bosch JM, Verzijlbergen FJ. Imaging the inflammatory activity of sarcoidosis: sensitivity and inter observer agreement of (67)Ga imaging and (18)F-FDG PET. *Q. J. Nucl. Med. Mol. Imaging.,* 2011;55:66-71.

In: Medical Imaging
Editors: M. D'Elia and A. Madaffari
ISBN 978-1-62081-049-1

Chapter 4

Analytical and Numerical Methods for Anatomical and Metabolic Medical Imaging

Francisco Malano*[1,2] *and Mauro Valente*[1,2]
[1] CONICET, Buenos Aires, Argentina
[2] Universidad Nacional de Córdoba, Ciudad Universitaria; Argentina

Abstract

There are several methods largely implemented and employed for daily medical imaging aimed to non-invasive early prevention and/or disease diagnosis.

This chapter is dedicated to radiological techniques in medical imaging. It concerns the interaction of ionizing radiation with patient. From a general point of view, it may be possible to characterise radiological medical imaging techniques in two different categories, the first one devoted to structural information to get anatomical images, whereas there are other type of methods dedicated to obtain functional information in order to provide some metabolic patient characterization.

It has been previously presented by several authors that this kind of imaging techniques may be suitably modeled and eventually improved by means of both theoretical and experimental approaches.

This chapter will concentrate on analytical along with corresponding numerical models, both integrated in dedicated algorithms capable

*E-mail address: valente@famaf.unc.edu.ar

of handling main physical phenomena related with radiation transport and interaction processes. Detailed description will be presented about the main features regarding radiation transport modeling for radiological purposes. As example, the developed medical imaging approaches will be implemented and preliminary tested for conventional absorption contrast anatomical imaging, like radiography, mammography and computed tomography (CT), as well as functional imaging methods like single photon emission computed tomography (SPECT).

PACS 87.57.-s, 87.55.kd, 87.55.K-

Keywords: Medical Imaging, Monte Carlo methods, Algorithms

AMS Subject Classification: 94A08, 65C05, 68W25

1. Introduction

In 1895, while Wilhelm Konrad Röntgen was experimenting with cathode tubes, he discovered that a fluorecent screen began to glow when it was struck by ligth emitted from the tube. He also observed that this effect remains even when he placed different objects between tube and screen. This led him to realize that the tube was emitting not only ligth, but should also be there another kind of radiation. He called it *X-radiation* or *X-ray* to signify an unknown type of radiation. Further experiments led him to observe that different materials attenuate X-ray of various ways, and that these rays could be recorded on a photographic film [1]. A few months later radiography was first used in clinical practice, and that was how began the medical imaging [1], [2]. After that, great efforts have been made to improve the quality and reliability of the results obtained in medical imaging techniques. Implementation of tomographic reconstruction applied to conventional radiography techniques led the way to what became known as Computed Tomography (CT) [3]. In parallel, although based on completely different physical principles, the appearance of Magnetic Resonance Imaging (MRI) provides another kind of information that complements CT, expanding the capabilities of medical imaging.

Nowadays, medical imaging includes a wide range of different imaging techniques, some of them considered invasive [1], such as endoscopy, and other considered to be non-invasive, like X-ray radiography, computed tomography, ultrasound, positron emission tomography, magnetic resonance, etc.

It is well known that early diagnosis may be the best strategy for non-invasive disease detection, significantly helping for treatment modality decision. Medical imaging constitutes a valuable method for this purpose, as well as suitable tool for contributing to disease treatment once visualized within human body. In this way, radiological medical imaging techniques are largely and worldwide implemented, aimed to non-invasive early prevention and/or disease diagnosis. From a general point of view, it may be possible to characterize radiological imaging techniques in two different categories: one devoted to acquire anatomical images, containing structural information, and the other dedicated to obtain functional information providing metabolic patient characterization [4]. Tomographic acquisition and subsequent reconstruction applied to conventional radiological imaging techniques provides a significant improvement to information contained in images.

It has been previously presented by several authors [5] [6] [7] [8] that radiological imaging techniques may be suitably modeled and eventually improved by means of both theoretical and experimental approaches.

This chapter will concentrate on analytical along with corresponding numerical models, both integrated in dedicated algorithms capable of handling main physical phenomena related with radiation transport and interaction processes [2]. Detailed description will be presented about the main features regarding radiation transport modeling for radiological purposes. As application examples, the developed models for medical imaging simulation will be implemented and preliminary tested for conventional absorption contrast anatomical imaging, like Computed Tomography, as well as functional imaging methods, like Single Photon Emission Computed Tomography (SPECT) [9].

1.1. Fundamentals of interaction of photons with matter

Throughout history, the wave-particle behavior of electromagnetic radiation has been a challenge for science. Nowdays, it is well known that photons can be thought as a zero rest mass and zero charge particle, whose energy E and momentum $\vec{p}$ are related to a wave of frequency ν by the expressions

$$E = h\nu \qquad \vec{p} = \frac{h\nu}{c}\hat{i}$$

where $c = 299792.458\frac{Km}{s}$ is the speed of ligth in vacuum, $h = 6.6256 \times 10^{-34} J \cdot s$ is Plank's constant and $\hat{i}$ is the direction of movement.

Since photons carry energy and momentum, they will be able to interact with other particles, such as electrons, protons, positrons, etc. Because they are electrically neutral, they do not continuously lose energy via coulombic interactions with atomic electrons as do charged particles. In fact, they travel long distances (compared with the distances traveled by charged particles) before having an interaction, and this interaction takes place when photons are very close to the other particle. This distance traveled without interaction is called *free path*. When an interaction takes place, photons can transfer a part, all or none of its energy to other particles. If a photon transfers all its energy, then it disappears and the strucked particle gains almost all the energy and momentum of the photon. The lack remaining energy is transferred to other particles, which are in most cases atoms. When photons transfer only a part or none of their energy, they and other particles may suffer scattering. The scattered angle of both particles is such that obeys conservation laws of energy and momentum.

In radiological imaging, photon beams are used to extract information from inside the human body. So, in this case, it is clear that photons interact with other particles that are arranged in form of atoms. As it is known, atoms consist of a very small positive charged nucleus surrounded by a negative charged cloud of electrons, sorted in *atomic levels*. Given that the nucleus is screened by electrons, photons mainly interact with the electronic cloud. However, interaction with the nucleus has a smaller but non-zero probability of occurrence, and this probability increases as the impinging photons energy increases. When performing radiological images, photon beams are usually employed with energy ranging from $30keV$ (mammography) up to $400keV$, approximately. High energy (often called "hard") photons can be emmited by some radioisotopes utilized to acquire metabolic images. In those ranges of energy, there are several ways in which photons can interact with particles or atoms:

- **Photoelectric effect**

  An electron bounded to its nucleus with energy E_b can be ejected if incident photon energy E_γ holds that $E_\gamma = h\nu > E_b$. In this interaction the impinging photon transferes all its energy, thus it disappears. Since conservation laws of energy and momentum forbid that a photon can transfer all its energy and momentum to a single electron, the greatest part of the photon energy goes to the ejected electron, and the remaining fraction to the atom as a hole, making the presence of the latter essential for the occurrence of this effect. That is why a bounded electron is extrictly necessary for a photoelectric effect to take place. The maximum possible energy of ejected electron is given by:

$$E_{e^-}^{max} = h\nu - E_b$$

where E_b is usually named *work function*. Once the interaction is carried out, the atom remains in an excited state in which one electron is missing. This missing electron is called a *vacancy* and an atom in this state is said to be *ionized*. This vacancy is quickly filled through the capture of a free electron from the medium and/or rearrangement of electrons from other shells of the electronic cloud. In either of these two cases, the electron occupying the vacancy must cede some of its energy to enter in the atom or for rearrange in atomic shells. This energy is emmited in form of *characteristic photons*, and the frequency of them depends exclusively of the difference of energy between shells (Figure 1).

The photoelectric effect requires photons with energies from a few electronvolts for atoms with lower atomic number Z, to over $1MeV$ in heaviest elements. For atoms present in biological tissues, which are of relatively low atomic number, photoelectric effect is the predominant interaction for impinging photons with energies between $10eV$ to $35keV$, approximately (refer to Figure 4 below).

- **Photoexitation**

  When the energy of the photon is not enough to eject electrons from the atom but this energy is exactly the necessary to elevate electrons from a shell to another, then the photon is entirely absorbed by the electron followed by a jump from its original shell to another in which its energy difference match the energy of the impinging photon. Subsequent relaxation of this state occurs emitting one or more characteristic photons, as is shown in Figure 1.

- **Incoherent scattering**

  Incoherent scattering, commonly named *Compton scattering*, happens when an impinging photon interacts with a free electron or with an atomic electron whose bounding energy is much lower than the energy of the photon:

$$E_b << E_\gamma = h\nu$$

  Due to this fact, direction of movement of both photon and electron change a given angle and a fraction of energy is transferred from the photon to the electron, as shown in Figure 2.

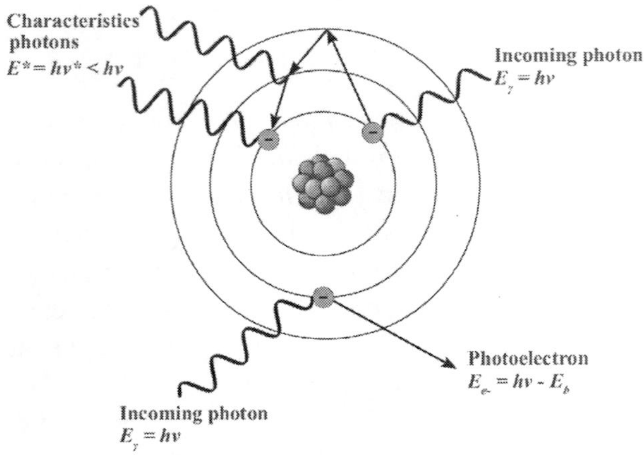

Figure 1. Photoelectric effect and photoexcitation followed by a relaxation scheme.

Applying the conservation laws of energy and momentum, it can be proved that the energy of the scattered photon is given by:

$$E'_\gamma = \frac{E_\gamma}{1 + \frac{E_\gamma}{m_0 c^2}(1 - \cos\theta)}$$

where E_γ is the energy of the impinging photon, m_0 is the rest mass of the electron and θ is the scattering angle. In the same way, energy of the scattered electron is given by:

$$E_{e^-} = \frac{E_\gamma(1 - \cos\theta)}{\frac{m_0 c^2}{E_\gamma} + 1 - \cos\theta} = \frac{2\cos^2\phi}{2 + \frac{E_\gamma}{m_0 c^2}\sin^2\phi + \frac{m_0 c^2}{E_\gamma}}$$

For biological tissues, this interaction is predominant between photon energies from $40keV$ to $1.2MeV$, approximately.

- **Coherent scattering**

  This kind of interaction, often referred to as *Rayleigh scattering*, is given between an impinging photon and the atom as a hole. In order to consider that atoms may behave as single entities, the energy of photons must be much smaller than the binding energy of electrons, that is $E_\gamma << E_b$. Impinging photons do not lose energy, only changing their movement direction.

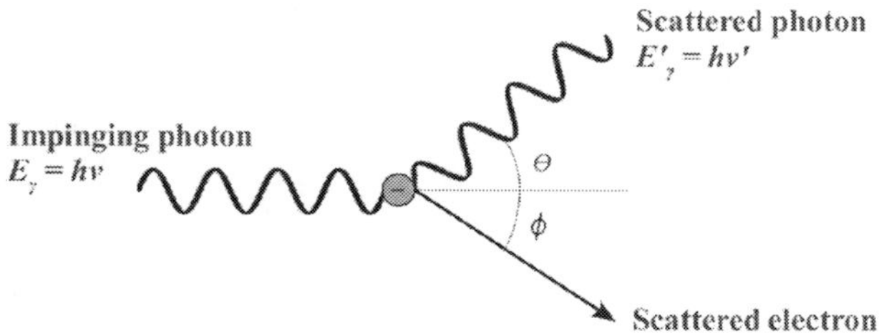

Figure 2. Photon (θ) and electron (ϕ) scattered angles.

The scattered angle is in average small for high photon energies and atoms of low Z, and this angle increases for lower photon energies and atoms of higher Z. For biological tissues and photon energies used in radiological imaging, coherent scattering is a relatively unlikely effect.

For impinging photon energies greater than $1.022 MeV$ there is another possible kind of interaction called *pair production*, in which a photon moving near an atomic nucleus can disappear causing a creation of a pair electron-positron. It will be not presented detailed discussion for that interaction since photons of this energetic range are usually not utilised in most radiological images. However, for Positron Emission Tomography (PET) imaging systems it is relevant to understand this process and even more its inverse process called *electron-positron annihilation*. For a detailed description of pair production and annihilation refer to specific bibliography, like [6], [10] and [11].

1.1.1. Cross section and Mass attenuation coefficient

As stated, photons can interact with particles in several ways and these interactions have certain probabilities of occurrence. Explanations will be presented considering homogeneous particle beams composed by $J = N/(S \cdot t)$ particles per unit area and time that impinges in a thin foil of width dx made of a certain material as shown in Figure 3. Assuming that an ideal detector is placed to count only outcoming particles that had not interacted with the foil. Then, the measurement recorded by the detector would be $J_{det} = J + dJ$, where dJ indicates the number of particles that effectively interacted with the foil. Observe that dJ must be a negative number, given that it considers the differences between outcoming and impigning particles.

It is easy to figure out that the beam is attenuated in targets represented by circular area (disc) where a certain amount of beam particles interact. These

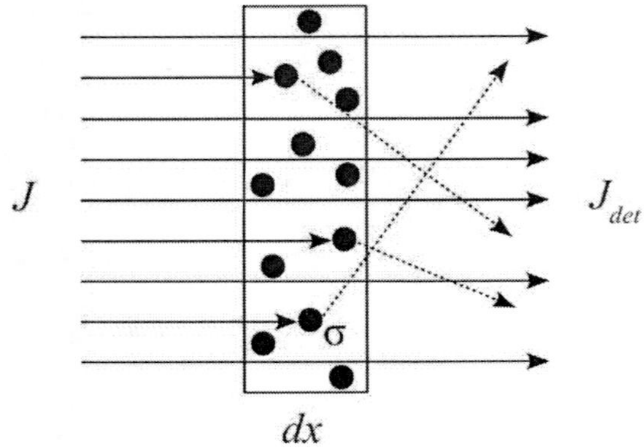

Figure 3. Atenuation of a homogeneous beam through a thin material foil.

discs or *scattering centers* can be thought of as representing atoms, molecules or other particles that compose the material foil. Since the beam is uniformly distributed over all the incidence area S, and the foil is considered of a differential width dx, the area fraction covered by target discs over the total incidence area is equal to the number of interacting particles over the total number of impinging ones. This could be mathematically expressed as follows:

$$\frac{dS}{S} = \frac{J - J_{det}}{J} = \frac{-dJ}{J}$$

where dS is the area covered by scattering centers and S is the total irradiation area. If σ is the cross-sectional area of a single scattering center, and dn_c is the number of scattering centers contained in a volume dV then

$$\frac{dS}{S} = \frac{dn_c\,\sigma}{S\,dx}\,dx = \frac{dn_c}{dV}\,\sigma\,dx = \eta\,\sigma\,dx \quad \Longrightarrow \quad \frac{-dJ}{J} = \eta\,\sigma\,dx \tag{1}$$

where $\eta = dn_c/dV$ is the number of scattering centers per unit volume. Particularly, in case of material with density ρ and molar mass M, it can be obtained

$$\eta = \frac{N_A\,\rho}{M} \tag{2}$$

where $N_A = 6.02214 \times 10^{23} mol^{-1}$ is the *Avogadro constant.*

It should be remarked that the number of interacting particles is directly proportional to σ, and this magnitude is intrisically related to the scattering center itself, independently of the density of scattering centers in the medium, since this latter is given by η. Due to its importance, σ receives the name of *cross section*, and it is proportional to the probability of interaction of a particle with the associated scattering center.

As discussed above, a particle may interact by several ways with a scattering center. It is natural to associate a particular cross section to each interaction type, where the sum of all particular cross sections results in the *total cross section* (σ_T):

$$\sigma_T = \sigma_{Photoelectric} + \sigma_{Compton} + \sigma_{Rayleigh} + \cdots$$

The total cross section, then, is related to the total probability of interaction, regardless its type. Figure 4 presents, as example, the water cross section for main types of interaction in the considered energy range. Calculating by

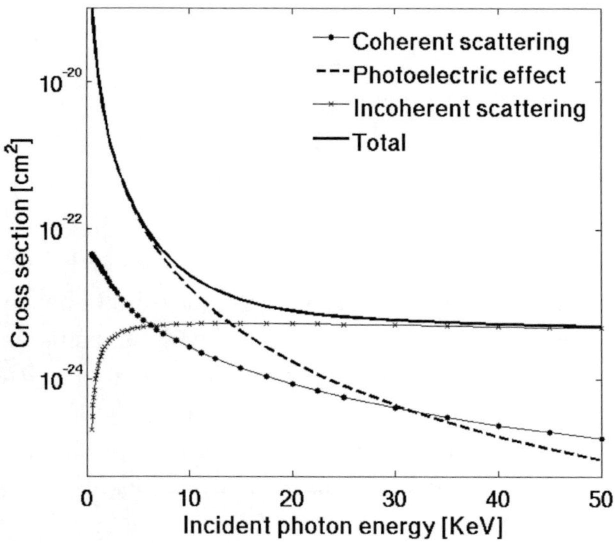

Figure 4. Water cross sections for different main interactions.

(1) the number of outcoming particles $J(L)$ that get through a foil of a non differential width L without interaction, should be obtained the following:

$$\frac{dJ}{J} = -\,\eta\,\sigma_T\,dx \quad \Rightarrow$$

$$\int_{J_0}^{J(L)} \frac{dJ}{J} = \int_0^L -\eta\,\sigma_T\,dx \quad \Rightarrow$$

$$\ln\left(\frac{J(L)}{J_0}\right) = -\eta\ \sigma_T\ L \quad \Rightarrow$$

$$J(L) = J_0 \cdot e^{-\eta\sigma_T L} \tag{3}$$

In some cases, it is useful to introduce new magnitudes called *attenuation coefficient* (μ) defined by:

$$\mu = \eta \cdot \sigma = \frac{N_A\ \rho}{M} \cdot \sigma$$

and *mass attenuation coefficient* (μ/ρ) given by:

$$\frac{\mu}{\rho} = \frac{N_A}{M} \cdot \sigma$$

Thus, it is clear that

$$\mu_T = \mu_{Photoelectric} + \mu_{Compton} + \mu_{Rayleigh} + \cdots$$

and by (3)

$$J(L) = J_0 \cdot e^{-\mu_T L} \tag{4}$$

It is important to realise that in a real detector, the number $J(L)$ of particles predicted by (4) will be always less than the measured one, since, besides of counting the particles getting through the foil without interacting, it also takes into account some particles scattered (photons scattered by Compton effect, for example). In many applications the scattering signal is low enough and can be neglected, but when a higher measurement precision is needed, this signal needs to be filtered with collimators or a post-process to reduce the noise caused by scattering.

1.2. General overview of Monte Carlo methods

Monte Carlo is a non deterministic or statistical method used to approximate mathematical expressions complex and expensive to compute. The method has its origin around 1944, as a research tool for development of atomic bomb during World War II, in Los Alamos National Laboratory (U.S.). In this work was done the probabilistic simulation of hydrodynamics problems concerning the distribution of neutrons in the fusion material, which has essentially a random behavior. The method name was given after the Casino of Monte Carlo (Monaco) because the roulette a simple generator of random numbers.

The Monte Carlo method is a powerful tool in many fields of mathematics, physics and engineering [12]. It is widely used to solve those problems for which deterministic algorithms would be extremely inefficient or impractical. Although it is true that it produces approximate solutions, one of the major advantages of this method is that it can be always possible to control the accuracy of those solutions in terms of the statistical error [12], [13]. If the problem is well posed, then the solutions satisfy the Central Limit Theorem [14]. So, if more presicion is desired, then more calculations are needed.

In many Monte Carlo applications dedicated to calculate physical phenomena, most processes can be directly modeled from known probability density functions (PDFs) for each particular event. This type of calculation is often called *Monte Carlo simulation*, because it tries to emulate as similar as possible what happens in reality. Simulation studies have several advantages over experimental ones, given that every simulation parameter can be changed in order to investigate the effect of each of these parameters on the system performance [12], [15].

Nowadays, Monte Carlo methods have won much ground in different areas, strongly reinforced by the development of modern computers, and particulary by parallel computing systems, which offer countless possibilities to improve the computation time [12].

2. Applications of radiation transport methods for medical imaging

This section is dedicated to show the suitability and potentiality of radiation transport modeling for its application on medical imaging fields.

All imaging techniques based on ionizing radiation, like X-ray beams, can be studied and modeled by means of the presented methods. Of course, it may be necessary to develop and implement dedicated adaptations for each one of the desired specific applications [1], [2].

This section includes explanations for general purposes guidelines along with some examples for anatomical and metabolic imaging techniques. In this framework, radiation transport is calculated including both complete and approximated solutions with the aim of remarking necessity and/or convenience of each of the modeling methods [2].

2.1. Modeling anatomical imaging techniques

Anatomical imaging methods generally employ external X-ray beams performing irradiation modalities aimed to get structural information. In this sense, patient anatomy may be obtained by means of these methods.

From a general point of view, typical anatomical medical imaging techniques consist on external X-ray sources generating radiation from the Bremsstrahlung of electrons reaching the anode constituting the target. Once radiation emerges from patient after interaction processes, its detection is performed by means of dedicated detectors (originally radiographic films and more recently improved devices like solid state detectors). Radiation detection is further traduced in the corresponding image, which may be hardcopy or analogical/digital format.

Therefore, the main features and required information to be included for anatomical imaging process modeling are the following:

- irradiation arrangement specifying facility configuration along with localization of patient and equipment components.
- precise knowledgement about spectral and geometrical characteristics of incident radiation beam.
- information about detector characteristics, general design details, radiation response, calibration, etc.
- patient or phantom anatomy from which material properties will be inferred.
- radiation-matter interaction models, which may be assessed by means of analytical expressions and/or tabulated parameters, like interaction cross sections.

Radiation interaction with patients can be interpreted as combination of two different contributions. The first one represents the so called primary component and it takes into account contributions from incident photons that do not interact with the patient. On the other side, the secondary component corresponds to contributions arising from scattered radiation generated by interactions of incident beam and patient anatomy. Characteristics of each one of these components are strongly dependent on the specific imaging modality and selected irradiation configuration. In addition, component importance and relevance can be suitably estimated and approximated according to involved physical parameters.

Accordingly, the guidelines described below are presented illustrating how to proceed with the most commonly used anatomical imaging techniques. Application results and analysis are used to assess the corresponding qualitative and quantitative performances of the implemented methodology.

2.2. Digital radiography

Nowadays, modern technology offers the possibility of digital systems for projection radiography. Digital radiography (DR) consists on patient planar projections generated when irradiating with conventional X-ray tubes. Radiation field size and orientation can be arbitrary selected and detection is performed by means of X-ray to visible photon conversion. Fluorescent or phosphorescent scintillator materials are used to convert, almost linearly, incident X-ray to visible ligth, which is further detected with some typical photographic device, like charge-coupled device (CCD) detectors or modern solid state detectors like flat panels. High performance of associated dedicated electronic system becomes also a main requirement.

Radiation source produces polyenergectic spectrum consisting on both Bremsstrahlung and characteristic photoelectric emissions. Besides, X-ray beam emerges from machine with geometric divergence affecting image detection.

Clinical radiographic equipments operate between 100 and 300kV, approximately. Due to typical thicknesses at different locations of the patients' body, it becomes necessary to have radiation transmission from 20 or even more centimeters of nearly water-equivalent materials. In this sense, primary component results the main, and actually almost all, contribution to radiation reaching the detector. This fact arises from the significant differences in energy hardness between primary and scattered components. It can be proved that scattering contribution to emerging radiation may be almost negligible, because its low energy spectrum. In addition, the air path between patient and detector gives an extra obstacle to the scattering component transmission required to reach the detector. Furthermore, usually detector sensibility does not present the same response and corresponding efficience for detecting photons having different energy. Actually, radiographic detectors sensitivity is typically optimized for assessing relative best efficiency at high energy X-rays and low efficiency for low energy photons; thus limitating scattering contribution to acquired images.

With the considerations explained above, it becomes acceptable to introduce the following approximation for the physical radiation transport in the framework of radiographic imaging:

$$I(i,j) = I_0(i,j)\, e^{[-\mu_{abs(E)}\, \rho\, z]} \tag{5}$$

where $I_0(i,j)$ and $I(i,j)$ state for the incident and emerging[1] intensities at the (i,j) pixel corresponding to specific detector location; whereas $\mu_{abs}(E)$ is the linear mass absorption coefficient evaluated at the corresponding energy, ρ is the material mass density and z is the traveled absorption frequency of this path. The extension to polyenergectic beams is easily accomplished by adding weighted components of the spectrum.

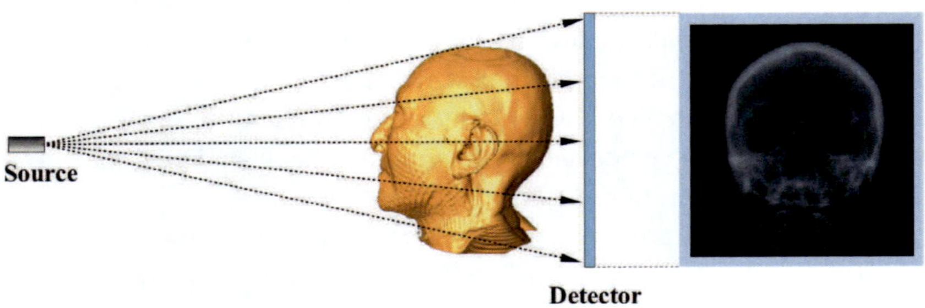

Figure 5. X-ray radiography irradiation setup.

The expression above applies to primary radiation component and does not take into account image contribution corresponding to scattering effects. However, the simplicity of this equation allows to implement analytical approaches for determistic calculation of radiation transport. This characteristic evidences the main reasons for the mentioned proposal. Otherwise, if all scattering effects need to be considered it becomes mandatory to compute complete radiation transport, which requires stochastic approaches except for extreme simple and typically useless configurations.

Figure 5 sketches the arrangement used for deterministic digital radiography calculation. X-rays beam emerges from a divergent source having energy distribution according to typical beams of clinical digital radiography X-ray spectra.

[1]strictly, it referes to radiation reaching detector

A dicom formatted real patient computed tomography (CT) has been used as irradiated sample for deterministic DR computation. As a first approach and with the aim of pointing out relevant features in simplified conditions, all the voxels corresponding to internal patient structures have been set as water-equivalent. The required adaptation for computing DR considering heterogeneous media can be implemented by means of suitably image segmentation based on Hounsfield index vs. relative electronic density CT calibration. Figures 6 and 7 report the obtained DR image and central profiles, respectively, by means of deterministic approach for both homogeneous and heterogeneous phantoms. The considered source-phantom distance was large enough for assuming that incident beam is quite similar to a parallel beam.

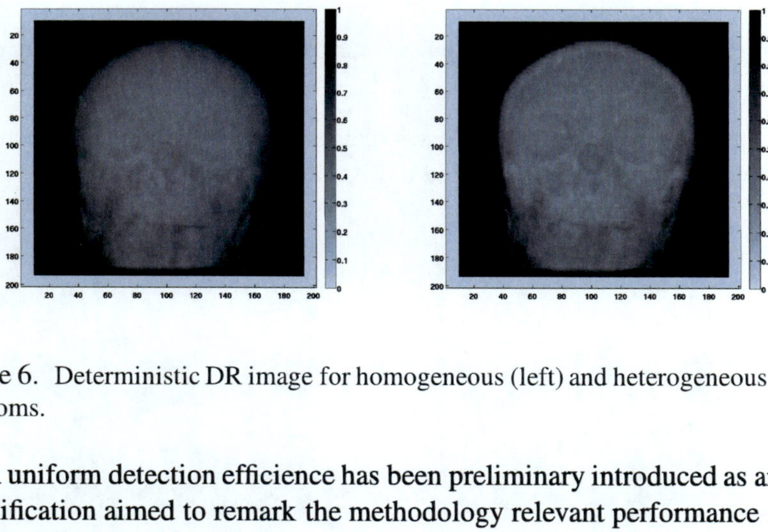

Figure 6. Deterministic DR image for homogeneous (left) and heterogeneous (right) phantoms.

A uniform detection efficience has been preliminary introduced as another simplification aimed to remark the methodology relevant performance avoiding unnecessary extra complications. Generalization for the inclusion of detection efficience can be easily accomplished assigning to each pixel a constant dependent upon specific pixel response and incident energy channel.

As mentioned, contrary to deterministic approaches, full stochastic radiation transport is capable of complete description of radiation-matter interaction processes, therefore providing both primary and scattering contributions. Coupled photon-electron full radiation transport has been implented by means of developed Monte Carlo simulation routines based on the general purposes PENELOPE [10] main code. Dedicated code routines have been developed to suitable handling of space voxelization as required for dicom CT informacion. Exactly the same calculations done with deterministic approach have

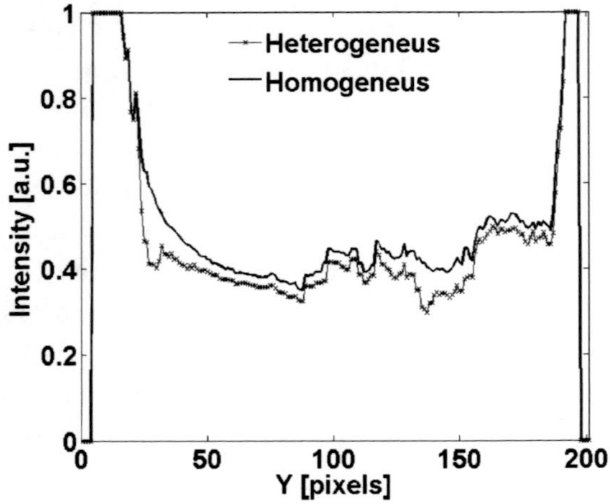

Figure 7. Profiles through central vertical axis for both deterministic images.

been repeated using Monte Carlo simulations [15]. The obtained results for DR image and profiles are reported in Figures 8 and 9; respectively.

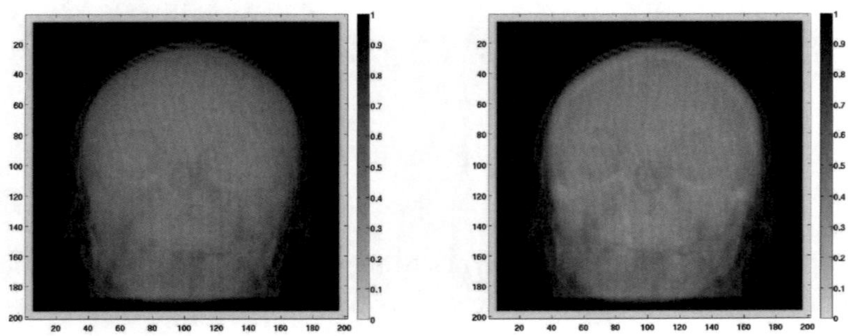

Figure 8. Stochastic DR image for homogeneous (left) and heterogeneous (right) phantoms.

Additionally, differences between stochastic and deterministic approaches were quantified as shown in Figure 9.

2.3. Mammography

Nowadays, mammography screening is a commonly used radiological technique dedicated to breast examination. Actually, a mammogram is usually

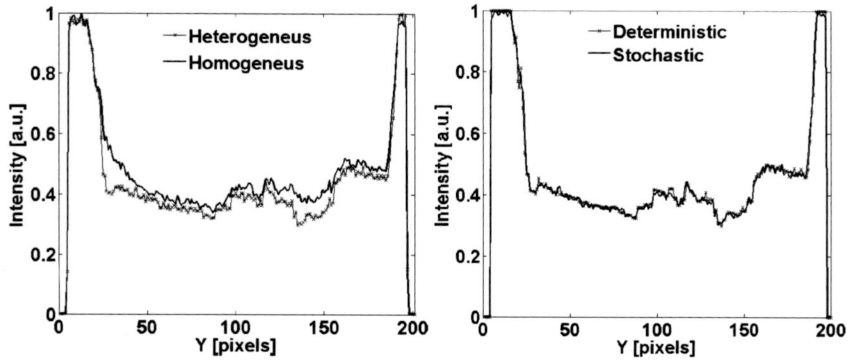

Figure 9. Profiles through central vertical axes from stochastic (left) and comparison between stochastic and deterministic heterogeneus (right) images.

recommended for women with the aim of assessing early detection and further diagnosis of breast deseases [1]. Typical clinical uses of mammography diagnosis is the evaluation of patients that may present some abnormal clinical findings [16], like breast lumps or cysts. Diagnostic mammography is also performed if previous screening mammogram showed abnormal details. In these cases, mammography screening is mainly concentrated around the region of interest.

Modern digital mammography (DM) consists on a mammography system but replacing traditional X-ray film by solid-state detectors [2]. Digital mammography, which was developed in part to overcome some limitations of traditional X-ray film based mammography, is capable of separating image acquisition and display therefore allowing their optimization.

Conceptually, mammography technique and associated equipment do not differ very much from DR. Actually, modeling both the imaging methodologies consists on the implementation of similar irradiation conditions and configurations. A simplified typical mammography configuration is sketched in Figure 10.

The designed breast sample in Figure 10 includes some details in order to mimic typical breast deseases. Just to point out how to proceed, microcalcifications (μCa) have been selected as breast details. Spatial distribution of μCa within breast volume has been taken as all of them were align along the longitudinal axis. Absolutely, any other desired configuration can be simply implemented. Radiation source was practically considered as an X-ray point source emitting photon distributed according to a typical mammogra-

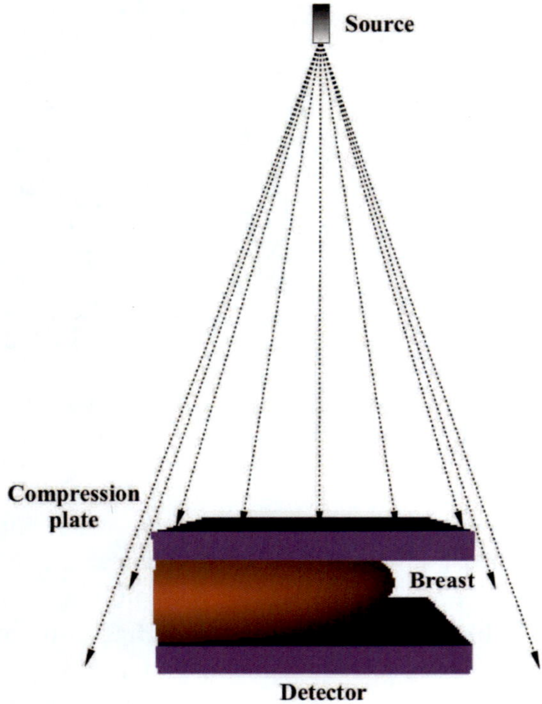

Figure 10. Sketch of simulated mammography irradiation setup.

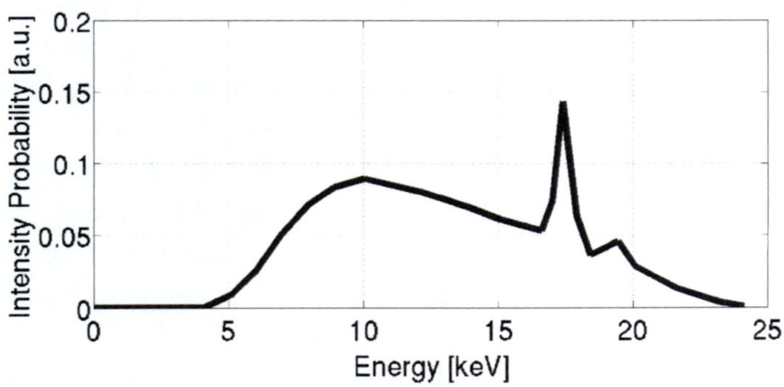

Figure 11. Example of mammography beam spectrum (25kV Molibdenum anode).

phy facility spectrum [7], [17]. The presented example corresponds to a 25kV Mo spectrum, as shown in Figure 11. Beam divergence was incorporated as geometrical divergence according to typical mammography equipments and screening configurations.

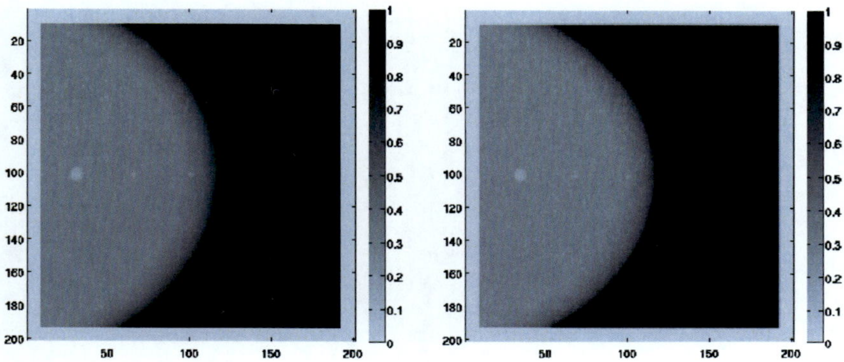

Figure 12. Deterministic (left) and stohastic (right) mammography image.

Radiation transport was performed assuming soft tissue as homogeneous material for the breast; whereas calcium oxalate was the choice for all μCa. In addition, radiation detection was performed assuming ideal detector. However, as mentioned for DR, it does not represent hard efforts to introduced specific detection sensitivity or efficiences.

Figures 12 and 13 report the obtained results for breast deterministic and stochastic mammography images and central profile comparison; respectively.

2.4. Computed Tomography

From a general point of view, computed tomography (CT) is a nondestructive powerful technique capable of producing bidimensional (2D) as well as tridimensional (3D) cross-sectional images of the irradiated sample [3]. The 3D sample reconstruction is actually obtained from typical flat X-ray projection images [1]. In this sense, internal structure characteristics, like sample dimensions, shape, and density can be assessed with CT techniques. Figure 14 shows a simplified sketch of CT set up including all relevant features of typical CT systems.

As shown in Figure 14, sample is placed on a turntable platform located between the radiation source and the image recorder system. Computed controlled devices are incorporated with the aim of assessing correlation of X-ray image acquisition with sample position (actually orientation). In this sense, typical 2D planar images are detected at each sample orientation. Finally, dedicated mathematical algorithms included in automatized software allow to

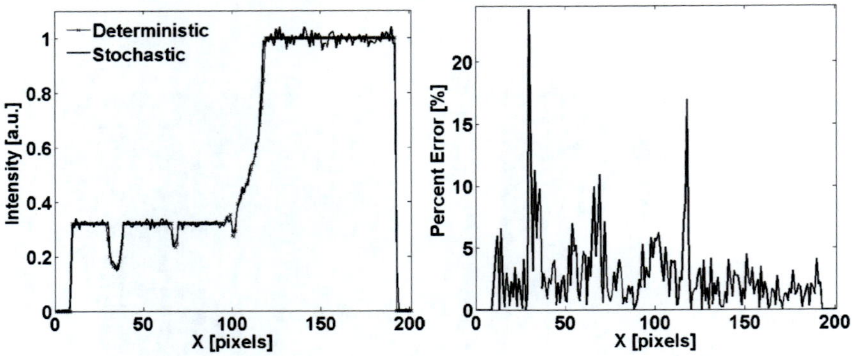

Figure 13. Central axis profile comparison (left) and corresponding differences (right).

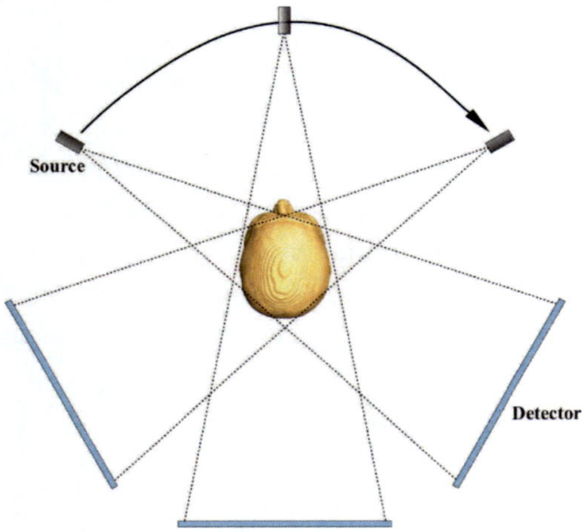

Figure 14. Sketch of CT irradiation setup.

achieve cross-sectional sample images from which 3D reconstruction can be directly performed.

Almost from the original development, CT technology and associated facilities have been rapidly implemented for medical imaging purposes. In fact, nowadays CT is one of the more important tools in daily medical imaging, because of its capability of improving conventional 2D X-ray radiography.

In the implemented methodology CT scanning was modeled by means of dedicated sample rotation algorithms. All collected projection images were stored for further processing. The typical tomographic reconstruction algorithm backprojection with Shepp-Logan filtration [3], [8], [18], [19] was incorporated to the calculation system in order to achieve sample cross-sectional images along with 3D volumetric reconstruction. As preliminary evaluation of the developed imaging systems, to study the performance of deterministic and stochastic approaches considering simple phantoms was convenient. This previous investigation is particularly useful for pointing out relevant features, preliminar performance and eventually non negligible limitations associated with the proposed approaches.

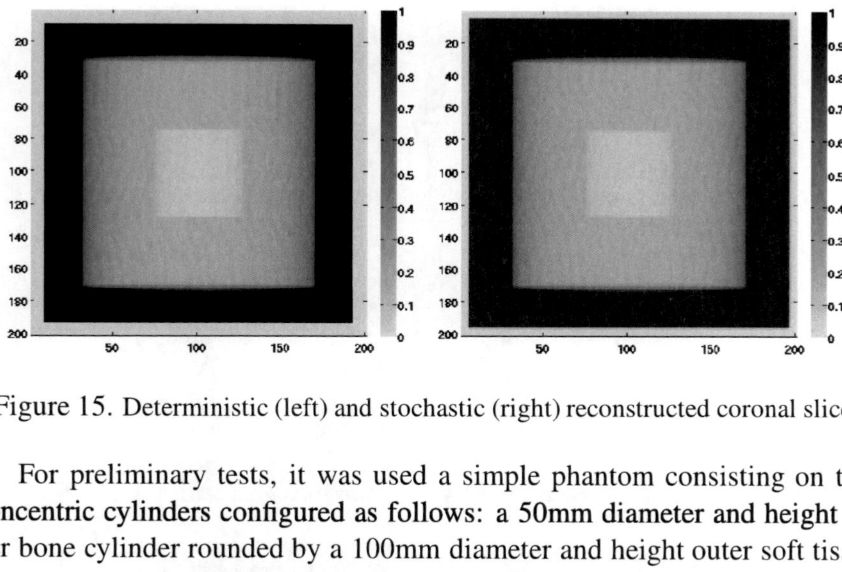

Figure 15. Deterministic (left) and stochastic (right) reconstructed coronal slice.

For preliminary tests, it was used a simple phantom consisting on two concentric cylinders configured as follows: a 50mm diameter and height inner bone cylinder rounded by a 100mm diameter and height outer soft tissue cylinder. Figures 15 and 16 present the obtained central coronal plane and corresponding profiles; respectively, for deterministic and stochastic reconstructed cross-sectional images.

Besides, the implemented tomographic reconstruction algorithm was carefully investigated profiting the suitable advantages of the deterministic approach. In this sense, CT reconstruction was performed changing the number of acquired irradiation projections. Figure 17 shows how the quantity of acquired projections influences the final performance of the CT method.

Once preliminary tests showed consistency of the proposed methods suggesting their reliability, it was considered a more realistic and demanding scenario consisting on a dedicated anthropomorphic heterogeneous phantom, as presented in Figure 18.

Figure 19 shows some typical reconstructed images at different slices.

Once CT slices are obtained it becomes direct to assess the corresponding

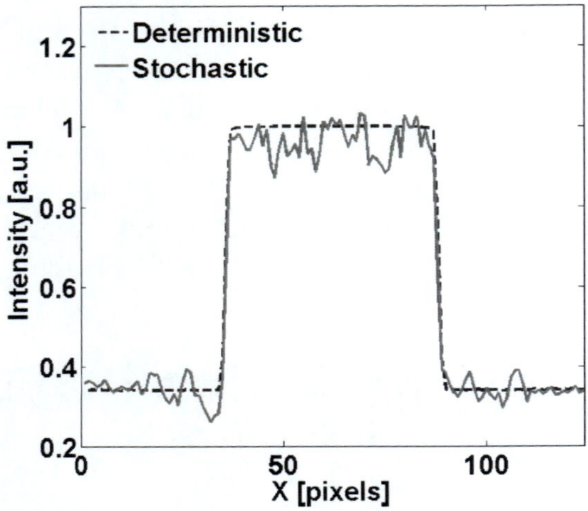

Figure 16. Deterministic (solid ligth) and stochastic (dashed dark) reconstructed image central profiles.

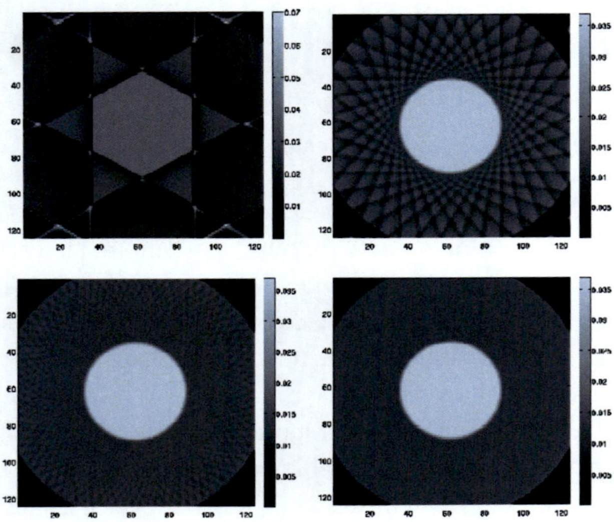

Figure 17. Reconstructed CT image using 3 (up left), 18 (up right), 45 (bottom left) and 180 (bottom right) projections.

phantom/patient volumetric reconstruction.

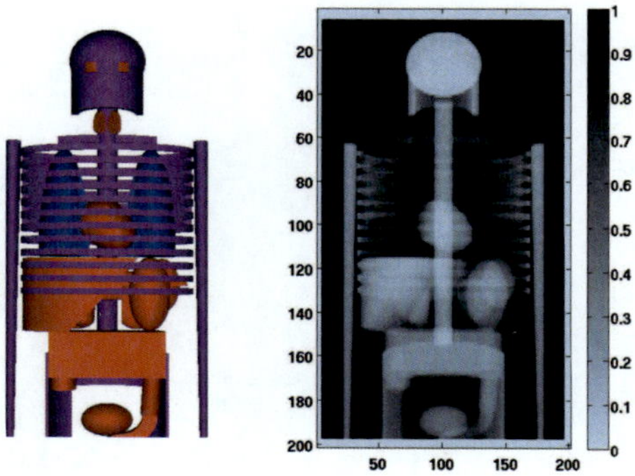

Figure 18. Designed anthropomorphic phantom for CT investigations (left) and corresponding DR (right).

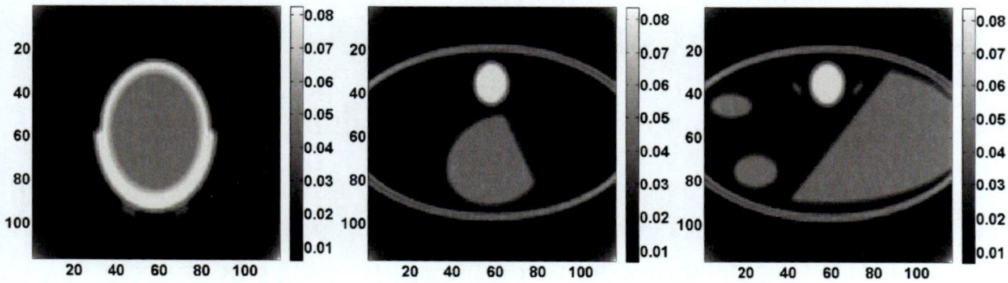

Figure 19. Slice label 25 in head zone (left), 100 at chest zone (middle) and 125 in abdomen zone (right) of dedicated anthropomorphic phantom.

2.5. Detector response incorporation

All application examples presented above were realized considering "ideal" radiation detection. However, particle counting instruments are made of gas, solid or liquid. Then, the passage of ionizing particles through detector sensitive material results in energy dissipation by means of ionization bursts, which are further converted into electrical pulses measurable with readout devices.

This section is dedicated to illustrate simple mechanisms for incorporating specific detector response. The proposed method consists on extremely oversimplified models, due to the fact that the only aim is to illustrate how to include better approaches for detection processes.

The method consists on incorporating specific detector response, mainly focused on energy efficiency but all other detection characteristics could be similarly considered. In this sense, typical medical imaging detectors were included in the developed radiation transport models. As example, knowing NaI

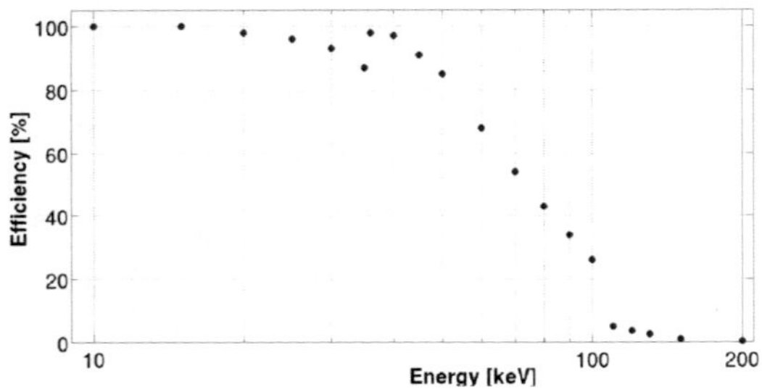

Figure 20. Efficiency for 1mm NaI.

detector efficiency, as shown in Figure 20, it becomes possible to introduce this information into the simulation codes, both deterministic and stochastic in order to assess better detection characterization.

2.6. Example for modeling metabolic imaging

Metabolic Imaging consists on combining medical image modalities with the use of some radiotracer with the aim of revealing physiological activities within patients for nuclear medicine purposes [9].

The traditional functional imaging technique is the gamma or Anger camera based on the detection of gamma photons by crystals in the camera detector, like sodium iodide. Gamma photons generated by radiopharmaceutical decay and leaving the patient are further counted at detection crystals that scintillate responding to the incident photons [15].

The first test for the developed radiation transport system in nuclear medicine was to perform gamma camera imaging. The obtained results, considering a simplified condition of a ^{99}Tc point source within a 3D dicom patient phantom, are shown in Figure 21.

2.6.1. Single Photon Emission Tomography (SPECT)

The aim of this section is to show general guidelines for the implementation of calculation models dedicated to assess, approximately, radiation transport in Single Photon Emission Computed Tomography (SPECT). Basically, the SPECT technique uses a gamma-emitting radioisotope injected into patient bloodstream [9], [20].

The injection of marker radioisotopes is performed with the objective of binding it to some radioligand, which has particular chemical binding proper-

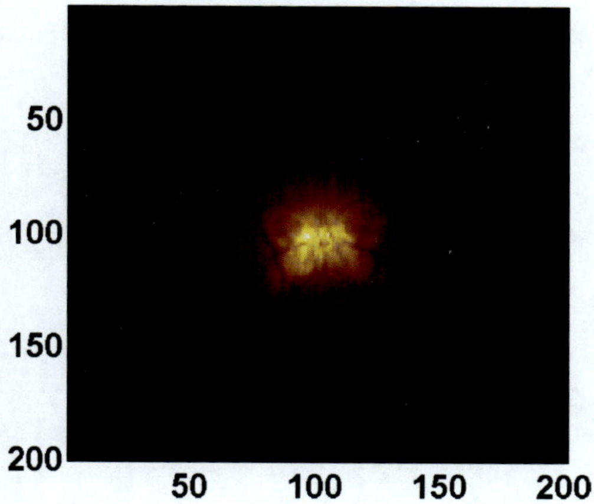

Figure 21. Gamma camera functional image corresponding to a point source inside virtual patient.

ties for specific biological tissues. Therefore, once radiopharmeceutical is already bound to a certain tissue, it becomes possible to detect the localization of the emitting source, which is correlated with the corresponding tissue [15].

In this sense, one of the most simplified ways to implement approaches capable of qualitatively achieving some of the main features of SPECT imaging is to consider a gamma-emitting source located at certain patient positions and/or within specific organs. Radioisotopes emission characteristics can be obtain from well known tabulated data in literature.

Both developed deterministic and stochastic radiation transport methods for generic metabolic imaging are capable of arbitrary defining radioisotope type along with location within patient anatomy. Therefore, it is possible to define the desired activity and/or irradiation time in order to generated the corresponding SPECT image associated with gamma rays emerging from patients' body and properly reaching radiation detectors.

One important feature of metabolic imaging techniques is detector designs. Specifically, collimator properties play a crucial rol in determining reliability and quality of recorded images. In this sense, it should be remarked that implemented approaches both deterministic and stochastic are suitable for further incorporation of specific user desired detector characteristics. In spite of that, but looking for simplicity the presented results refer to "ideal" detection, *i.e.* no specific detector was incorporated therefore meaning that only direct almost parallel rays are recorded at each detector pixel.

Figure 22 reports the obtained tomographically reconstructed central plane SPECT images by means of deterministic approach.

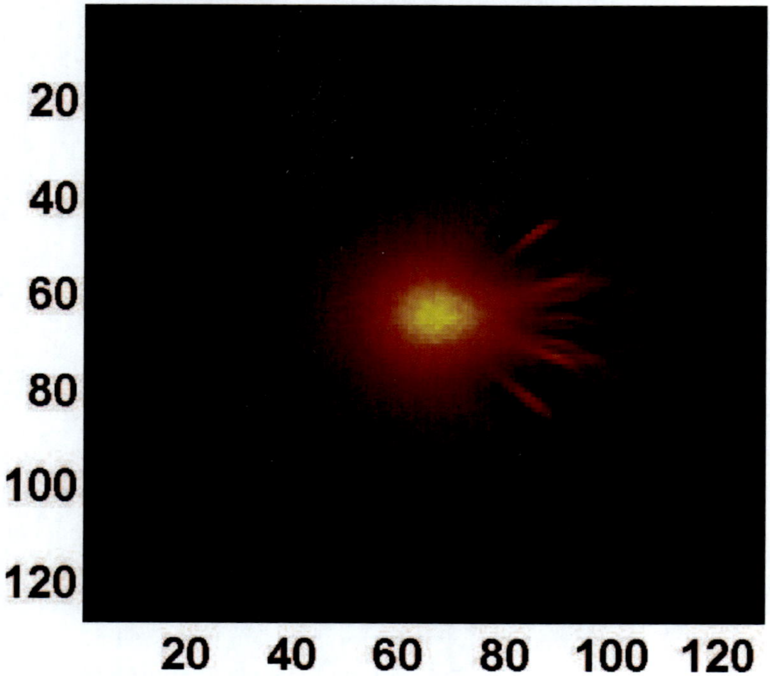

Figure 22. Deterministic SPECT image slice (head region) for a point ^{99}Tc source inside virtual patient (a) and corresponding SPECT-CT wavelet fusion (b) by means of stochastic approach.

Aditionally and finally, Figure 22 also shows the corresponding SPECT-CT fusion achieved by means of wavelets fusion algorithms [8] applied to a virtual patient CT and SPECT images both obtained with stochastic approach.

Inherent image matching is achieved due to the intrinsic spatial correspondence between implemented anatomical and metabolic imaging methods, regardless of deterministic or stochastic approaches. Therefore simplifying further image processing like SPECT-CT fusion. In the example presented above, fusion process was performed by wavelets theory, but the developed imaging system allows the user to select other mechanisms according to the convenience for each case.

3. Conclusion

This work has shown practical and simple procedures for radiation transport modeling applied to medical imaging. It has been proved that the proposed methods based on both simplified deterministic and full stochastic approaches were feasible. Furthermore, it was possible to implement both the methods in different medical imaging techniques even when considering anatomical and metabolic imaging.

3.1. Radiation transport models

Radiation transport has been modeled by means of different approaches, clearly conceptually distinguishable one from the other. The first approach consisted on oversimplified models focused on overall medical imaging description. The developed mechanism was to implement a ray-tracing method limitating radiation transport just to computing primary beam component disregarding absolutely scattering processes within sample and associated contributions to the recorded signal. This approach even if based on oversimplified approximations has demonstrated to provide good enough capability for qualitative purposes. In addition, once validated against reliable methods the deterministic method may be useful to investigate the effect of some imaging parameters, like beam spectrum, beam divergence, sample characteristic and associated transmission, etc. Its capability for performing imaging within microseconds, *i.e.* almost immediate, should be pointed out as the main and remarkable advantage of the deterministic method. This characteristic constitutes a really valuable tool for preliminary investigations about medical imaging dependence upon setup configuration, as mentioned above.

On the other hand, the developed Monte Carlo method for radiation transport modeling in medical imaging procedures was based on full radiation transport description by means of solving numerically Boltzmann radiation transport equation. This approach allows to consider absolutely all physical processes involved in radiation transport as well as radiation interaction within the sample and detector devices. Radiation matter interaction can be performed in base of analytical models and tabulated data for double differential cross sections. The implemented method obtains the corresponding interaction probabilities from the main code PENELOPE, whose theoretical models and tabulated data are absolutely and largely validated.

3.2. Image formation and detection physics for anatomical and metabolic imaging

The obtained deterministic images have been calculated using simple ray-tracing mechanims with associated effective path attenuation within the sample. The implemented method was to consider a ray coming out from point or extended sources and following up its trajectory to each detector pixel. In this framework, source-sample-detector attenuation paths were calculated according to the effective linear mass attenuation coefficient in correspondence to the geometrical trace from the source to each one of the detector pixels. Therefore, by computing traveled distance it was possible to assess fluence transmission across samples.

Contrary, the Monte Carlo method allowed to compute absorption contrast images by means of completely following emitted particles step-to-step calculating at the end of each track the corresponding eventual changes of phase space variables, like energy loss, movement direction, etc. In this framework it is possible to have primary particles not arriving at the detector or even more they can leave the considered "simulation universe". Additionally, all eventually generated secondary particles need also to be considered up to their absorption or when they leave the user defined "simulation universe". In this sense, it becomes possible to have secondary radiation contributions to the detected image, which produces typical image blurring and sometimes distortions. It should be emphasized that this fact is obviously present in real imaging processes.

Finally, it is appropriate to mention that detector response can be included in both the developed imaging approaches by means of suitable description that may significantly improve imaging capture by specific detection devices. It was not the aim of this work to study in depth this feature, but general guidelines have been provided.

3.3. Final remarks about the implemented radiation transport models

First of all, it should be stressed that different radiation transport models were proposed as approaches for medical imaging purposes. It has been proved that both of them can be successfully implemented by theoretical frameworks as well as the corresponding automatized calculation systems.

The simpler method consisting on the approximation of neglecting scattering processes has shown to be easy to implement due to the possibility of using almost directly the well known ray-tracing mechanism. In this sense, the implemented deterministic approach consists on a suitable but critical approximation of the complete Boltzmann equation neglecting diffusive terms associated to scattering processes. Therefore, it results in solving a linear first order differential equation for radiation fluence from which the well known Lambert-Beer law is obtained for describing primary radiation attenuation.

Main limitations of the deterministic method correspond to the lack of scattering consideration. No radiation matter interactions are computed, except for effective attenuation of primary particles, therefore avoiding its application for reliable quantitative characterizations. On the other hand, relevant advantages of the deterministic approach are its simplicity providing quick image computation capable of acceptable qualitative description of general imaging features.

Main advantages of the developed Monte Carlo simulation subroutine for complete radiation transport modeling derive from the obtained significant improvement in comparison with the deterministic approach. This method allows to assess both mean values and corresponding uncertainties for imaging. The inclusion of interaction processes within irradiated sample as well as conside- rations of specific detector material and structure contribute to the reliability of this method providing more realistic imaging description. Therefore, the obtained images can be appropriately compared with real medical images, even from a quantitative point of view. The inherent stochastic nature of Monte Carlo methods implies that significant computation resources will be necessary requiring more calculation time than deterministic approaches. A characteristic of the implemented Monte Carlo method is its capability for computing real full radiation transport obtaining accurate description for both primary and scattering contributions. One disadvantage may be the large computation times that are required to be spent for accurate (good enough) statistical precision.

The developed and implemented methodologies for medical imaging characterization have demonstrated to be valuable tool for virtual imaging investigations. Preliminary, the obtained results show good qualitative and quantitative agreement when compared with real medical images. Further investigations are still necessary for achieving definitive conclusions.

Final conclusions are that the proposed method could be suitably transfered to routine clinical practice, for example to obtain digital reconstructed radiography (DDR) in radiotherapy treatment planning or study possible equipment-patient setup configurations for optimizing image quality according to the specific imaging parameters involved in the desired technique.

References

[1] I. Bankman. *Handbook of medical image processing and analysis.* ElSevier Academic Press, California, 2009.

[2] Seibert A. Leidholt E. Boone J. Bushberg, J. *The essential physics of medical imaging.* Lippincot Williams and Wilkins, 2001.

[3] T. Buzug. *Computed Tomography.* Springer-Verlag, 2008.

[4] P. Suetens. *Fundamentals of Medical Imaging.* Cambridge University Press, second edition, 2009.

[5] P. Duvauchelle, N. Freud, V. Kaftandjian, and D. Babot. A computer code to simulate x-ray imaging techniques. *Nuclear Instruments and Methods in Physics Research B,* (170):245–258, 2000.

[6] S. España, J. L. Herraiz, E. Vicente, J. J. Vaquero, M. Desco, and J. M. Udias. Penelopet, a monte carlo pet simulation tool based on penelope: features and validation. *Phys. Med. Biol.,* (54):1723–1742, 2009.

[7] G. Tirao, C. Quintana, and M. Valente. Mammography image quality optimisation: a monte carlo study. *Int. J. Low Radiation,* 7(4):276–297, 2010.

[8] C. Epstein. *Introduction to the mathematics of medical imaging.* Siam, Philadelphia, 2003.

[9] G. Saha. *Physics and radiobiology of nuclear medicine.* Springer-Verlag, 2006.

[10] J.M. Fernández-Varea, J. empau and F. Salvat, S.; Fernández-Varea. PENELOPE-2008: *A Code System for Monte Carlo Simulation of Electron and Photon Transport.* Nuclear Energy Agency, Barcelona, Spain, 2009.

[11] F.H. Attix. *Introduction to Radiological Physics and Radiation Dosimetry.* Wiley-VCH, 1987.

[12] S Dupree and S. Fraley. *A Monte Carlo premier.* Kluver-Plenum, New York., 2002.

[13] P. Bevington and D. Keith Robinson. *Data reduction and error analysis.* McGraw Hill, 2003.

[14] H. Tijms. *Understanding Probability: Chance Rules in Everyday Life.* Cambridge University Press, 2004.

[15] M. Ljungberg, S. Strand, and M. King, editors. *Monte Carlo calculations in nuclear medicine: Applications in diagnostic imaging.* Institute of Physics Publishing, 1998.

[16] J. Ducote and S. Molloi. Scatter correction in digital mammography based on image deconvolution. *Physics in Medicine and Biology,* Vol. 55(No. 5):1295–1309, March 2010.

[17] C. Arvanitis and R. Speller. Quantitative contrast-enhanced mammography for contrast medium kinetics studies. *Physics in Medicine and Biology,* Vol. 54(No. 5):6041–6064, September 2009.

[18] A. Kak and M. Slaney. *Principles of Computerized Tomographic Imaging.* IEEE Press, New York, 2001.

[19] S. Bushong. *Computed Tomography.* Mcgraw-Hill, 2000.

[20] M. Stabin. *Fundamentals of nuclear medicine dosimetry.* Springer Science+Business Media, Spring Street, New York, NY 10013, USA, 2008.

In: Medical Imaging
Editors: M. D'Elia and A. Madaffari
ISBN 978-1-62081-049-1

Chapter 5

ELECTRICAL IMPEDANCE TOMOGRAPHY IMAGING: PRINCIPLES AND RECONSTRUCTION ALGORITHMS

Alancássio Eulálio[1,*]***, Leonardo R. F. Ribeiro***[1†]
and Wellington P. dos Santos[1,2‡]
[1]Universidade de Pernambuco, Brazil
[2]Universidade Federal de Pernambuco, Brazil

1. Introduction

In Recent years, Electrical Impedance Tomography (EIT) [1] has been used as a technique that could help health professionals to observe some human body structure behavior. Nowadays, Being EIT a non-invasive, non-radiating, non-ionizing and inexpensive methodology, it has been extensively studied in clinical diagnosis [4], biomedical engineering [5] and biotechnology [6]. Attempts are also being made to develop a better medical-EIT system for different clinical investigations and long time patient monitoring. Nowadays, applications do not care about images quality, because these applications are over working lungs, heart blood flux and, in these situations, there are no importance in determine a good image when reconstructed. In despite of that and

*E-mail: ae@ecomp.poli.br
†E-mail: leorfr@gmail.com
‡E-mail: wellington.santos@ufpe.br

how EIT is a low cost and a non-invasive technique [4], ones intend to use it for other medical approaches in order to provide a better image reconstruction quality. Although acquisition is reasonably simple, reconstruction EIT images is computationally a hard task, consisting in a numerical solution of Laplace's equation on specific grid of domain elements, using Finite Element Method (FEM), Finite Differences Method (FDM) and so on [12] [13] [14]. Also, image quality could be improved by a misfit of calculated and measured data in the reconstruction process, creating a error projection approach, called Projection Error-based Regularization (PEPR) method, necessary due to ill-poseness nature of EIT problem.

EIT reconstruction problem is an ill-posed one, that is, it has no only a unique solution. Numerical Methods of Laplace's equation solution result in smooth reconstructed images, this smoothness may be not interesting in medical applications, where is important well define features, as organs or tumors boundaries, for example. This chapter comes to introduce a purpose to obtain better results on image reconstruction, using an unsupervised classification technique plus quantization, based on Self Organizing Kohonen Maps (SOM) from reconstructed images by EIDORS (Electrical Impedance and Diffuse Optical Reconstruction Software), that is based in FEM numerical method of domain discretization associated with PEPR. That purpose, by an image pixels classification, define, through smoothness reduction of reconstructed image, a better image reading stronger associated with interest region within domain.

EIDORS is a reference tool in EIT image reconstruction research area and allows to create a comparison basis to new researches in EIT.

2. Electrical Impedance Tomography

At first, it is going to talk about EIT technique as itself. EIT idea comes from 1978, proposed independently, by Henderson and Webster [1]. Into several applications of EIT is highlighted, in this chapter, medical application that has been more and more used, because patients are not exposed to ionizing radiation and acquisition equipment require a very simple hardware architecture, furthermore there is a mobility feature in it allowing move equipment to patient. Electrical Impedance Tomography is a non linear inverse problem [8] in which the electrical conductivity distribution of a closed domain, in an object under test called phantom, [15] [16] is reconstructed from the surface potential at the boundary, developed by injecting a sinusoidal current signal [14]. A low frequency, from 10kHz to 1MHz, and low magnitude constant current is injected through an array of N surface electrodes, surrounding the domain to be imaged using different electrode switching protocols [5] and the boundary potentials are measured [14], although the boundary currents can also be measured for an applied voltage signal in Applied Potential Tomography [17]. The voltage data collected by the data acquisition system is then processed by an image reconstruction algorithm in a PC. Disadvantage from this technique is still associated with low resolution of reconstructed image.

After voltages on these electrodes were measured, it could evaluate a resistivities matrix and, after this, phantom of image could be determined by a certain iterative numerical method. The EIT problem could be divided in two different problems. First one is associated to domain discretization, named *direct problem*. To get that discretization, ones apply methods as FEM (Finite Elements Method), QM (Quadrangular Meshes), FVM (Finite Volume Method), TM (Triangular Meshes) and also is possible to mix methods each other [10] [11]. Each element from this discretization and its nodes allow to create a linear system of equations, which solutions provide *a priori* object, useful on the reconstruction step. Second EIT problem is called *inverse problem*, where from obtained voltages is possible to solve it by an iterative numerical method of Laplace's Equation solution, generating a phantom as close as possible that result established in direct problem solution. The inverse EIT problem has a high computational cost.

2.1. EIT Mathematical Modeling

In order to estimate the nodal potentials for a known conductivity, a relationship can be established between the electrical conductivity (σ) and spatial potential (Φ). Electrodynamics of EIT is governed by a nonlinear partial differential equation, called the Governing Equation [2] [3] of Electrical Impedance Tomography, which is given by:

$$\nabla.(\sigma\nabla\Phi) = 0 \tag{2.1}$$

It is possible to obtain a relation between the voltages measurements made on the domain boundary ($\partial\Omega$) and the domain conductivity, as follows:

$$\Phi = [K(\sigma)][I] \tag{2.2}$$

Where σ is elemental conductivity values, Φ is a vector of nodal potential and K is the transformation matrix, constructed from the elemental conductivities and nodal coordinates.

If K and I are known, (2.2) can be solved numerically using FEM to calculate the nodal potentials of the domain for the known conductivity (σ). It is known as the *forward problem*. Using the Gauss-Newton method [18] applied on EIT, the update vector of σ can be expressed as:

$$\sigma = [Q][\Phi_d] \tag{2.3}$$

Where Q is a function of the Jacobian matrix J and regularization parameters [19] [20]. Φ_d is the mismatch vector between calculated boundary potential (V_c) and measured boundary potential (V_m). That means if the matrix Q and the surface potentials Φ are known then the elemental conductivity (σ_e) can be mapped. This is called EIT *inverse problem* , which will be further discussed. Using the Modified Newton Raphson (MNR) iterative technique or any other, a suitably assumed conductivity vector (initial guess), $[\sigma_0]$ is modified to $[\sigma_0 + \Delta\sigma]$ for achieving a specified error limit in the calculated and measured voltage, updating the conductivity σ by a $[\Delta\sigma]$, obtaining $[\sigma_0 + \Delta\sigma]$.

2.2. Gauss-Newton approach: Image Reconstruction

Electrical conductivity imaging is a highly nonlinear and ill-posed inverse problem. The response matrix $[J^t J]$ is a singular matrix, that is, a matrix without inverse. In EIT, a minimization algorithm is used to obtain the approximate solution of the *inverse problem*. In order to get minimum solution, the object function, i.e, the difference between the experimental measurement data (V_m) and the computationally predicted data (V_c), is minimized. In inverse problems a least square solution [19] [20] of a minimized object function (s), widely used method, obtained from the calculated voltage data and the measured voltage data is searched by a Gauss-Newton method based numerical approximation algorithm is called the inverse solver. If V_m is the measured voltage matrix and f is a function mapping an N-dimensional (N is the number of elements in the FEM mesh) impedance distribution into a set of M (number of the measured data available) approximate measured voltage, then the Gauss-Newton algorithm works to find a least square solution of the function

(s) [19] [20] defined as:

$$\mathbf{s_r} = \frac{1}{2}||V_m - f||^2 + \frac{1}{2}\lambda||G\sigma||^2 \tag{2.4}$$

In (2.4), it has s_r how least-square error of reconstructions, G is a regularization parameter and λ is a positive scalar named regularization coefficient. (2.4) could be rewritten as:

$$s_r = \frac{1}{2}(V_m - f)^t(V_m - f) + \frac{1}{2}\lambda(G\sigma)^t(G\sigma) \tag{2.5}$$

Since for that, one differentiates it with respect to σ, obtaining one more simplified equation:

$$s_r{}' = -(f')^t(V_m - f) + \lambda(G)^t(G\sigma) \tag{2.6}$$

Where the term f' is equals to J, known as Jacobian matrix of size $g \times h$ and is defined by [20] as:

$$J = [f']_{gh} = \frac{\partial f_g}{\partial \sigma_h} \tag{2.7}$$

where $g = 1,2,3,\ldots,N$ (N = number of FEM elements in a grid),
$h = 1,2,3,\ldots,M$ (M = number of data measured per current projections (d) $\times$ number of current projections (p)).

By ill-posed nature of EIT, the $[f']^t$ matrix, in (2.6), is ill-conditioned which implies that just a small error on the measurement will make solution of (2.6) change strongly and is necessary a regularization term to make it well posed and it is incorporated to that equation. Differentiating (2.6), again, with respect to σ it reduces to:

$$s_r{}'' = (J)^t(J) - (f'')^t(V_m - f) + \lambda(G)^t G \tag{2.8}$$

By Gauss-Newton (GN) numerical method,

$$\Delta\sigma = -\frac{s_r'}{s_r''} = \frac{(J)^t(V_m - f) - \lambda(G)^t(G\sigma)}{(J)^t(J) - (f'')^t(V_m - f) + \lambda G^t G} \tag{2.9}$$

Neglecting higher terms, $\Delta\sigma$ reduces to:

$$\Delta\sigma = \frac{(J)^t(V_m - f) - \lambda(G)^t(G\sigma)}{(J)^t(J) + \lambda G^t G} \tag{2.10}$$

Replacing G^tG by I (identity) implies (2.10) as follows:

$$\Delta\sigma = \frac{(J)^t(V_m - f) - \lambda I\sigma}{(J)^t(J) + \lambda I} \tag{2.11}$$

To solve this problem by an iterative manner, the conductivity update vector of (2.11), in k^{th} iteration(k being a positive integer), must be reduced to:

$$\Delta\sigma_k = [[J_k]^t[J_k] + \lambda I]^{-1}[[J_k]^t(\Delta V)_k - \lambda I\sigma_k] \tag{2.12}$$

Thus the GN method based in inverse solver algorithm gives a regularized solution of the conductivity distribution for k^{th}-iteration as follows:

$$\sigma_{k+1} = \sigma_k + [[J_k]^t[J_k] + \lambda I]^{-1}[[J_k]^t(\Delta V)_k - \lambda I\sigma_k] \tag{2.13}$$

where $\mathbf{J_k}$ and $(\Delta V)_k$ are the Jacobian and voltage difference matrix respectively at the kth-iteration.

2.3. PEPR method

Although PEPR method is cited, in this chapter, as one way to improve the reconstructed image quality in EIT and the resistivity reconstruction is studied in EIDORS, it does not care about study it deeply. Generally, the choice of an appropriate regularization can be evaluated or found empirically [21] and the regularization parameter is related to an objective function [18]. The projection error could be utilized as the objective function; hence the regularization parameter would be expected to be related to the projection error. Furthermore, the value of regularization is required to vary with projection error. That is to say, a greater regularization value is needed for a larger projection error during iterations. If the projection error is very low, only a small regularization value is needed to regulate the ill-posed process [21].

In this section, it was observed a mathematical modeling of *inverse problem* solution using Gauss-Newton method, due to the fact to be used by EIDORS on its reconstruction works, as is going to be shown ahead, by an association of it with KSOM (Kohonen Self Organizing Maps) as a post-processing technique, in order to help health professionals on detection of interesting regions to be diagnosed. The PEPR method comes as an improvement of image quality by an insertion of a regularization parameter which varies according with error reduction along iterations, i.e, as higher is the error, implies either a higher regularization parameter while smaller is the error, smaller will be the regularization parameter as well.

3. EIDORS

EIDORS [9] [13] is an EIT- Electrical Impedance Tomography and Diffuse Optical (it still not implemented by EIDORS project) image reconstruction tool, whose objective is to provide an image reconstruction software that is freely modifiable and distributed too. EIDORS allows one constructs reference to form basis for new systems and methods, as well as allow new ideas are constructed and tested. As it is a freely modifiable code, EIDORS permit another researchers criticize and expand originals algorithms and their applications as well. First version of EIDORS was created in 2001 (version 1) and was based in Vaukhonen Thesis. Version 1 of EIDORS had consist in a MATLAB package, used to generate bidimensional grids, solve *direct problem* and exhibit images.

3.1. Software Architecture

Basically, EIDORS architecture could be described as a set of following software primary structures *data, image, fwd model* and *inv model*, and their combinations. Each of objects is represented by a structure. All of them have both name and type properties. The name property is arbitrary and is exhibited by graphics functions, which could be useful to distinguish from that ones specified by users. Type property is used to identify various objects categories(e.g. data, image, etc.) [9].

3.1.1. Fwd model

Is the most complex structure. Projected to represent Finite Element Model electrodes properties, positions and stimulation patterns, as well as pointers to the functions will solve *direct problem* in this model.

3.1.2. Data

The object *data* represents a measurements frame or simulated data. This structure require measurements fields, **meas**, and acquisition time, **time**, measured in seconds after each iteration. In a particular application one could consider, for example, **time** could be defined as related with another start point, as experiment start, or could be supposed 0 or -1 for unrecognized times or simulated data.

3.1.3. Inv model

This EIDORS object, join all necessaries informations to provide image reconstruction. There are two basic reconstruction types, based on **reconst type** field of this object, that is, **difference** one, which evaluate an image based in two data object and the **static**, which evaluate an image based on unique image.

3.1.4. Image

Image object contain simulated or reconstructed conductivities values. O **Elem data** ($N \times 1$) is the each value of image elements in the FEM in the field *fwd model*. For example, for a given object *inv model* called **imdl**, it could represent an image reconstruction by:

$$\mathbf{img} = \mathbf{invsolve}(\mathbf{imdl}, \mathbf{dado1}, \mathbf{dado2});$$

Similarly, in order to simulate a **data** object *datasim* from a certain image simulation *imgsim*, one could writes:

$$\mathbf{datasim} = \mathbf{fwdsolve}(\mathbf{fmdl}, \mathbf{imgsim});$$

In this chapter EIDORS was used to solve two different problems. First one is the *direct problem*, associated with diffusion elliptic equation solution, that governs electrostatic voltage distribution within a domain Ω and is given by (2.1).

Taking advantage from EIDORS functionality, there was made modifications in order to solve *direct problem* and generate figures which represents a solution. EIDORS uses a MATLAB package, as said before, to produce bidimensional meshes, based on FEM, solve *direct problem* and exhibit images. EIDORS was used to generate bidimensional meshes to solve three different direct problems, represented by three geometrical structures, a central circle, a lozenge and "malignant tumor". It will be shown bidimensional meshes that were generated to solve that three different models of *direct problem*, whose domain consists in objects where the impedance is considered to be double of background one. The domain reading were accomplished by external alternated currents patterns, through 32 electrodes, on domain boundary, disposed as regular manner and were imposed on them an opposite stimulation current pattern.

The second EIT problem to be treated by EIDORS the calculation of *inverse problem*, considered a ill-posed one, as said before, because internal potentials are extremely from domain impedances, as well as quantization errors, introduced by FEM and those associated measurement process [22].The inverse problem is solved by an iterative numerical method, by an objective function minimization, that is, the problem solution for an specific resistivities distribution of a certain domain [12]. EIDORS uses a non-linear regularized solver in order to find a unique and stable solution for an *inverse problem* [21]. The reconstructed images will be shown ahead. It was used the iterative Gauss-Newton method to reconstruct images establishing an approximation *difference*, from EIDORS, by Laplace's method. All results comes from simulation on EIDORS, version 3.4. As is possible to see in figures 1-6.

4. Kohonen Self Organizing Maps - KSOM

The Kohonen networks have biophysical inspiration. They are based on the brain functioning observations where the non-supervised learning is predominant. The Kohonen Self Organizing Maps are analogies to the logical structure of how the information is organized inside the brain [22]. Its main use is to group the inputs that have similarities among themselves creating classes or groups named clusters [23]. In general, the Kohonen SOM, can have one or two dimensions. Their learning strategy is based on competitive learning so there is a need of an objective function to define the winner neuron. One of the metrics there are most used is the Euclidean distance between the inputs (x_j) and the set of neurons weight (w_{ij}). This distance is defined by:

$$d_{xw} = \sqrt{\sum_{j=1}^{n} (x_j - w_{ij})^2} \tag{4.14}$$

After the winner neuron is calculated, its weights are adjusted by the com-

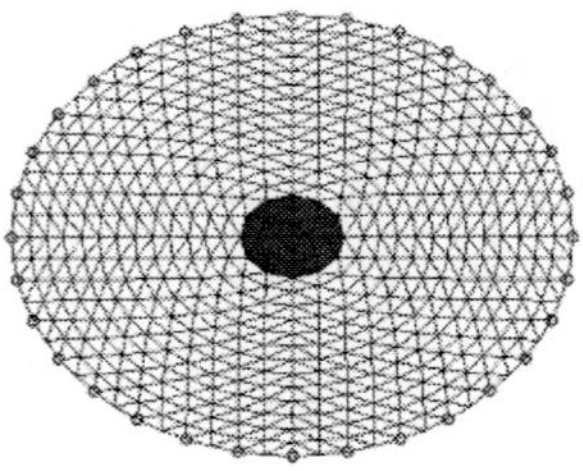

Figure 1. Central circle

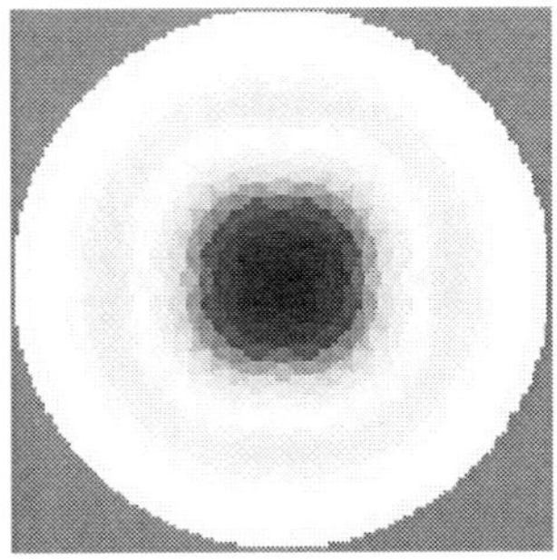

Figure 2. Circle image reconstructed by EIDORS

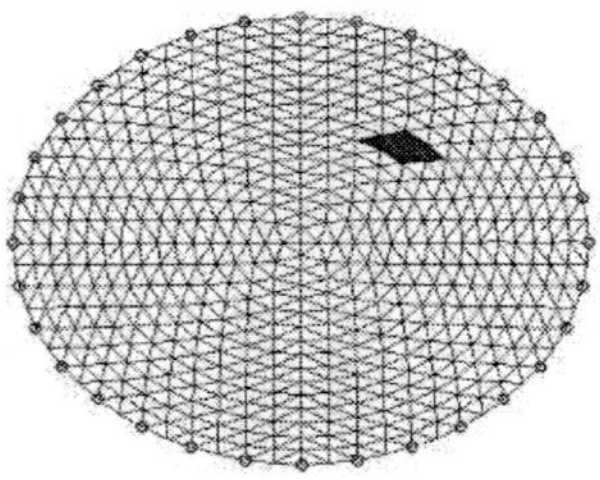

Figure 3. Lozenge image

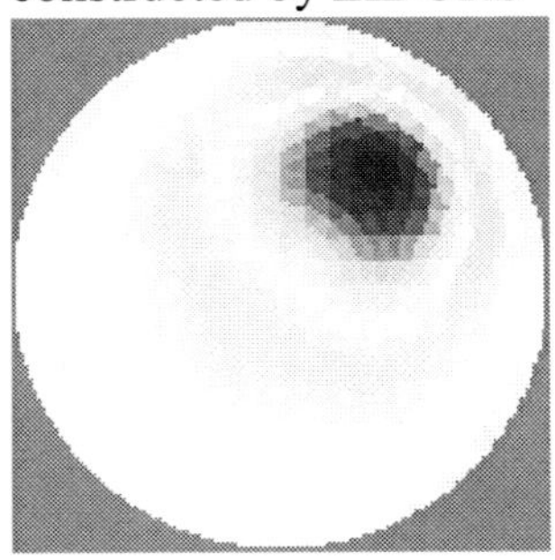

Figure 4. Lozenge image reconstructed by EIDORS

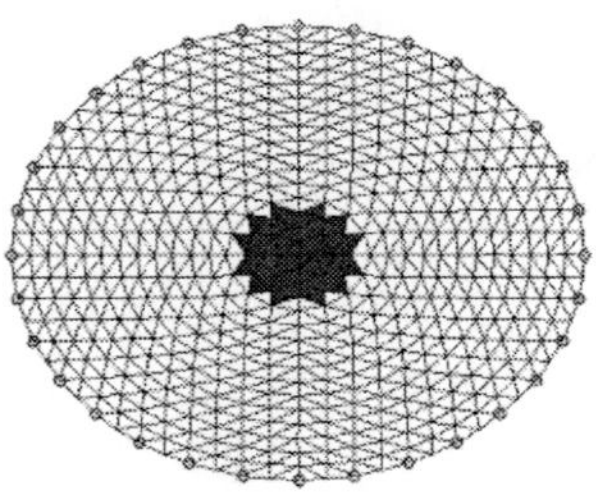

Figure 5. "Malignant tumor" image

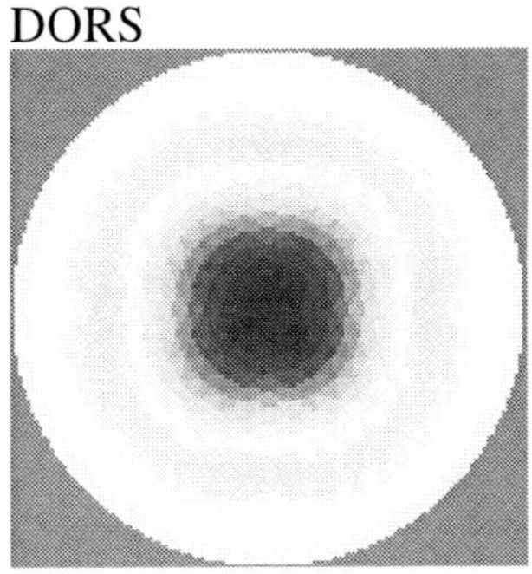

Figure 6. "Malignant tumor" reconstructed by EIDORS

petitive learning process adopted. There are two kind of competitive learning processes: the winner takes all or the winner takes quota. In the first one, only the weights of the winner neuron are adjusted. In the second one, the weights of the winner neuron neighbors are adjusted as well. The neighborhood of the winner neuron is established by the neighborhood function. One of the functions most used is the Gaussian function which creates a circular neighborhood region around the winner neuron. On this chapter, was used the winner takes all competitive learning process. The weights were adjusted in accordance with the following expression:

$$w_{ij}^{v}(t+1) = w_{ij}^{v}(t) + \alpha.(x_j - w_{ij}^{v}(t)) \quad (4.15)$$

Where w_{ij}^{v} are the synaptic weights that connect the input to the winner neuron, α is the learning rate and $x_j$are the inputs.

In order to obtain the results that will be presented. The learning rate was reduced at each iteration. The objective was to achieve a fine tuning and to try to avoid local minimal. At each iteration, the new learning rate was calculated by the following expression:

$$\alpha(t+1) = 0.9\alpha(t) \quad (4.16)$$

5. Application and Results

Allying this preceding technique to images produced by EIDORS, as shown in figures 1-6, it could be demonstrated a manner to concentrate health professionals attention on the interest region of a certain structure under analysis, by a classification and quantization of that images generated using EIDORS, with KSOM help. It will be observed that the results do not preserve the structure form, because this is not its characteristics, but clusterize similar elements on an image instead. So that is capable to focus where is more likely, find an interest object, in present case, is a region that posses a double of background impedance, as characterized in the section when was mentioned about EIT technique.

5.1. Technique Implementation

The code, used for clusterization and quantization of EIT images reconstructed by EIDORS figures 1-6, was edited in MATLAB environment. To construct that code were, used as input parameters, **Tapini** and **Nit**. As output parameter was used the variable **Nclusters**. That three images, generated by EIDORS, simulate an existence of a structure to be investigated using EIT technique. From that images reconstructed, were generated three test images denominated, respectively, *Central circle, Lozenge and "Malignant tumor"*, shown in figures 1-6. As shown in figure below, it was quantized each of test images and put each of them as inputs of KSOM code.

These quantized images were obtained by an iterative method over KSOM code for *Tapini* equals to 0.9, *Nit* equals to 150 and *Nclusters* equals to 5. In these figures were considered measurements from 32 electrodes, the reconstruction made by EIDORS using GN method of Laplace's equation solution(see EIT mathematical modeling) and then, it could be obtained all respective quantized images, as the best of them. It is possible, by figures examination, conclude that image reconstructed by EIDORS contains several smoothness on their boundaries turning difficult to define interest regions, alternatively one could percept a better boundary definition in quantized images offering a better condition to medicals diagnosis.

6. Conclusions

By the results demonstrated in previous section, it concludes that KSOM application allied with EIDORS tool, generate images with less smoothness, displaying to be possible isolate interest regions of image.

Clinically, KSOM application could help health professionals, once that resulting image could be quantized in a well defined boundaries, reducing medical professional observing area of structure to be diagnosed.

In this chapter, it was exposed only qualitative application in order to validate KSOM application in images EIT quantization [24], although could be used any metrics to analyze it as a quantitative manner. This metrics could be, for example, Retrieved Contrast Percentage (RCP), defined as difference between the mean of impedances from interest region of domain and mean of background region, of reconstructed image, divided by the difference between impedances mean of interest region of domain and the mean of impedances of background region, in the original image.

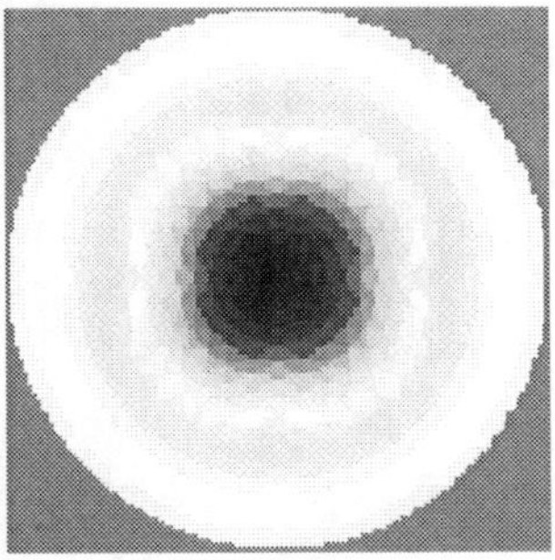

Figure 7. Central circle reconstructed

Figure 8. Quantized image

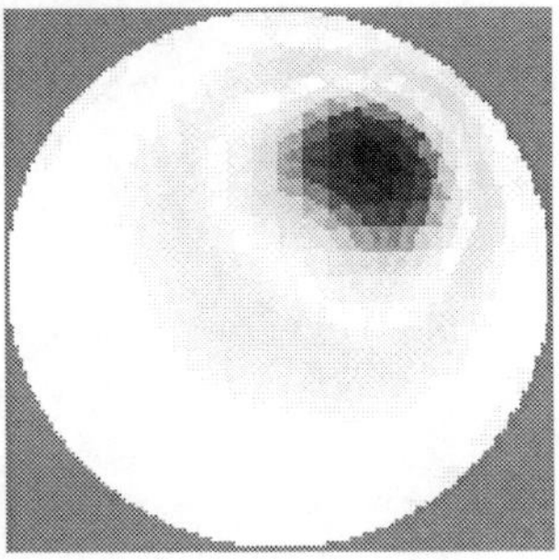

Figure 9. Lozenge reconstructed image

Figure 10. Quantized Lozenge image

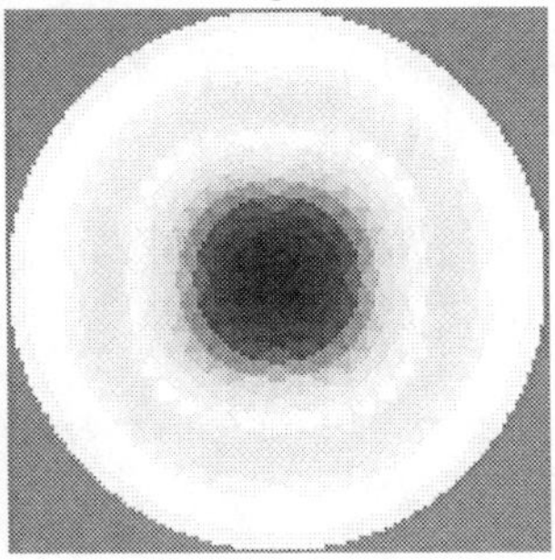

Figure 11. Reconstructed "Malignant tumor" image

Figure 12. Quantized "Malignant tumor" image

References

[1] Webster J.G. *Electrical Impedance Tomography*. Adam Hilger Series of Biomedical Engineering, Adam Hilger, New York, USA 1990.

[2] Denyer C.W.L. *Electronics for Real-Time and Three-Dimensional Electrical Impedance Tomographs*, PhD Thesis, Oxford Brookes University, January 1996.

[3] Metherall P. *Three Dimensional Electrical Impedance Tomography of the Human Thorax*, PhD Thesis, University of Sheffield, January 1998.

[4] Li Y., Rao L., He R., Xu G., Wu Q., Yan W., Dong G., Yang Q. *A Novel Combination Method of Electrical Impedance Tomography Inverse Problem for Brain Imaging*. IEEE Trans. Magnetics. 41(5):1848-1851, 2005.

[5] Brown B.H. *Medical impedance tomography and process impedance tomography: a brief review*. Measurement Science & Technology. 12:991-996, 2001.

[6] Linderholm P., Marescot L., Loke M.H., Renaud P. *Cell Culture Imaging Using Microimpedance Tomography*. IEEE Trans. on Biomed. Eng. 55(1):138-146, 2008.

[7] Hou W.D. and Mo Y.L. *Increasing image resolution in electrical impedance tomography*. Electronics Letters. 38:701-702, 2002.

[8] Lionheart W.R.B. *EIT reconstruction algorithms: pitfalls*, Review Article, challenges. Physiol. Meas. 25:125-142, 2004.

[9] Adler A. and Lionheart W.R.B. *Uses and abuses of EIDORS: an extensible software base for EIT*, IOP Publishing Ltd, 2006.

[10] Alves A.C. *Numerical Solutions Verifying of 2D Laplace's Equation by Multiples Richardson Extrapolations*. PhD Thesis. UFPR, 2010.

[11] Aguillar J.C.Z. *Numerical Studies on EIT Problems*. PhD Thesis. USP, 2009.

[12] Garnadi A.D. and Kurniadi D. *Two Dimensional Numerical Reconstruction of Electrical Impedance Tomography using Tikhonov Regularization*

Algorithms with a-posteriori parameter choice rule, IPB (Bogor Agricultural University), 2005.

[13] Lionheart W.R.B., Arridge S.R., Schweiger M., Vauhkonen M., Kaipio J.P. *Electrical Impedance and Diffuse Optical Tomography Reconstruction Software*, 1st World Congress on Industrial Process Tomography, Buxton, Greater Manchester, April 1999.

[14] Holder E.D. *Part 1 of Electrical Impedance Tomography: Methods, History and Applications*, p. 3-64, Institute of Physics Publishing, 2004.

[15] Bera T.K. and Nagaraju J. *A Stainless Steel Electrode Phantom to Study the Forward Problem of Electrical Impedance Tomography (EIT)*. Sensors & Transducers Journal. 104(5):33-40, 2009.

[16] Bera T.K. and Nagaraju J. *A Reconfigurable Practical Phantom for Studying the 2D Electrical Impedance Tomography (EIT) Using a FEM Based Forward Solver*, 10th International Conference on Biomedical Applications of Electrical Impedance Tomography, 2009, School of Mathematics, The University of Manchester, UK, June 2009.

[17] Brown B.H., Barber D.C., A.D. Seagar. *Applied potential tomography: possible clinical applications*. Clin. Phys. Physiol. Meas. 6:109-121, 1985.

[18] Biswas S.K., Rajan K., Vasu R.M. *Interior photon absorption based adaptive regularization improves diffuse optical tomography*, Proc. SPIE, Volume 7546, 2010.

[19] Graham B.M. *Enhancements in Electrical Impedance Tomography (EIT) Image Reconstruction for 3D Lung Imaging*, PhD thesis, University of Ottawa, April 2007.

[20] Yorkey T.J. *Comparing reconstruction methods for electrical impedance tomography*, PhD thesis, University of. Wisconsin at Madison, Madison, WI 53706, 1986.

[21] Niu H., Guo P., Ji L., Zhao Q., Jiang T. *Improving image quality of diffuse optical tomography with a projection-error-based adaptive regularization method*. Optics Express. 16(17):12423, 2008.

[22] Taner T. and Turham M. *Kohonen Self Organizing Networks with "Conscience"*, Rock Solid Images, 1997.

[23] Haykin S. *Neural Networks: A Comprehensive Foundation*, MacMilliam College Publishing Company, New York, 1994.

[24] Eulálio A., Ribeiro L.R.F., Valença M.J.S., Santos W.P. *Uso de Mapas Auto Organizáveis de Kohonen para quantização de imagens de Tomografia por Impedância Elétrica reconstruídas pelo software EIDORS*. X Congresso Brasileiro de Inteligência Computacional - CBIC, 2011, Fortaleza. Anais do X CBIC, 2011.

In: Medical Imaging
Editors: M. D'Elia and A. Madaffari
ISBN: 978-1-62081-049-1

Chapter 6

IMAGING OF BRAIN FUNCTION WITH POSITRON EMISSION TOMOGRAPHY AND ITS ROLE IN APHASIA RESEARCH

Wolf-Dieter Heiss*
Max Planck Institute for Neurological Research, Cologne, Germany

ABSTRACT

Positron Emission Tomography (PET) is at present the only method affording three-dimensional regional quantitation of various physiological, functional and molecular variables in man. Making use of tracers labelled with short lived positron emitting radio-nuclides and coincidence detection of annihilation radiation state of the art technology and advanced computing systems permit quantitative imaging of voluminous organs within one session. By 3-D data acquisition the distribution of small tracer amounts in the brain can be measured with a spatial resolution of down to 2 mm and values of various metabolic, functional and molecular parameters can be calculated applying kinetic and parametric analysis. Over the last 30 years PET has gained importance as a clinical diagnostic procedure yielding information on pathophysiologic mechanisms in various brain diseases. This method has also been used extensively as a tool of functional neuroanatomy when changes of metabolic or perfusional patterns were studied during various

*Tel: 49-221-4726-220 Fax: 49-221-4726-349, e-mail: wdh@nf.mpg.de

stimulations or task performances in healthy subjects or patients with localized brain lesions.

This approach was especially successful in the study of language, which as a complex brain function is based on the interplay of a distributed network in which partial functions are executed in various centres, which are hierarchically organized and lateralized into the dominant hemisphere. Following local brain lesions different language domains are impaired causing the various types of aphasia. Changes in the interactions within the functional network of language are important for the type of aphasia and for the capacity for recovery, e.g. after stroke. In this context, studies of activation patterns during speech tasks in the course after stroke could be used to predict extent of recovery, could demonstrate effects of supportive therapy and may be helpful in the development of procedures, e.g. cortical stimulation, for suppression of interfering or for enhancing compensatory effects in rehabilitation.

INTRODUCTION

The utilization of biological probes labelled with short lived radioisotopes makes positron emission tomography (PET) a powerful tool to image function, blood flow, metabolism, transmitter activity, receptor distribution, enzymatic activity, gene expression and other molecular variables in the brain. The high sensitivity allows PET to measure concentrations of molecules in the nano- or picomolar range without affecting the biochemical system being investigated. The wide versatility has made PET an important tool for experimental and clinical neuroscience. PET also played a pioneering role in analyzing the response of brain structures to sensory, motor and cognitive stimulations and thereby providing an insight into the functional organization of the intact brain and the compensatory mechanisms to lesions and diseases. In this context PET identified the various components of the functional network involved in speech perception and production and visualized the effect of damage of eloquent areas on activation patterns, which were also useful for predicting recovery and treatment effects in aphasia.

A SHORT HISTORY OF PET

Positron emission tomography is based on a group of artificial, cyclotron-produced radionuclides (e.g. ^{15}O, ^{11}C, ^{13}N, ^{18}F) with short half-lives and chemical properties permitting labelling of tracers relevant in biology and medicine. Therefore, compounds labelled with these radionuclides have been of interest for a long time, but received special attention when Ter Pogossian et al (1969, 1970 [1, 2]) performed the first quantitative measurements of regional cerebral blood flow (rCBF) and regional cerebral oxygen consumption ($rCMRO_2$). Positron-emitting radionuclides are characterized by an unique decay scheme: A positron is emitted from a labelled probe molecule, losing energy by collision with electrons in the tissue until within a very short distance (< 2 mm) it annihilates with one of these electrons. This annihilation converts the mass of the electron and positron into energy which is liberated in the form of two 511-keV gamma rays which are emitted in opposite direction. These gamma rays have sufficient energy to escape the body and can be detected by external detectors connected in and thresholded for "coincidence". By this "coincidence detection" the line along which the annihilation (and therefore the positron emission) took place can be determined. By combining lines of response from many different angles data can be reconstructed into cross-sectional images using mathematical algorithms. For the reconstruction of the distribution of a positron emitting radionuclide in a transverse section filtered back projection [3, 4] was developed. This formed the basis for the production of the first PET camera [5], an hexagonal array consisting of 64NaI crystals with photomultipliers and electronics connected in coincidence arrays. The first commercial one-ring camera, the ECAT II became available in 1978 [6] and was distributed to a considerable number of institutions interested in transferring the principle of quantitative tissue autoradiography for blood flow [7] and metabolism [8] to human brain research. Since the first proto-types (review in [9]) the technological advances of PET have been impressive (review [10]): Multiring cameras permitted simultaneous data acquisition from several brain slices and also allowed limited reconstruction in the axial direction [11]. New detector material (Bismuthgermanate, BGO, Lutetium orthosilicate, LSO) improved light yield and deadtime, new technology (segmented blocks of BGO or LSO detectors coupled to 4 photo multipliers, [12] or recently to avalanche photo diodes (APD) improved spatial resolution and permitted investigations of the whole brain in 3 dimensions with a spatial resolution of 2.5 to 5 mm [13, 14]. However, for a definite anatomic assignment of functional or metabolic values still coregistration to imaging modalities with high resolution of morphology, e.g. MRI, is necessary.

PET Scanners collect data by recording the coincidence combinations between opposing detectors. In order to increase counting efficiency the one-to-one coincidence coupling was soon replaced by a fan beam response from one detector to an array of opposing detectors in the image plane (ECAT II, [6] and with neighbouring rings for acquisition of inter-ring transversal images (e.g. PC-384, 4 rings for 7 slices, [11]). In modern PET scanners multiple rings of detectors allow simultaneous collection of multiple planes of images (e.g. ECAT EXACT HR, 47 slices from 24 rings, [13]). The sensitivity of scanners was further increased by 3 D data acquisition by which all gamma-ray pairs which intersect the PET scanner within a predefined response time are collected and used for reconstruction. Thereby the lines of response are tremendously increased – for the ECAT EXACT HR with nearly 20000 BGO detectors to many millions, for the HRRT with close to 120000 LSO elements to 4.486 x 10^9 possible lines of LORs [14]. – and the demands for computing power are accordingly high.

However, also by further increasing the number of detectors spatial resolution attainable with PET is limited [10]. The 180° emission of 511 keV gamma rays is not exact and this deviation impairs the exact localization of an annihilation event by 2 mm for a usual PET system. Before interacting with an electron the positron travels some distance, and the range depends on the energy with which the positron is emitted. The resulting degradation of spatial resolution is between 0.4 (^{18}F) and 1.5 mm (^{15}O). Fortunately, these errors are not additive but convolved together, and the resulting resolution limit is close to 2 mm, as it is already realized in high resolution tomographs for experimental [15] and human applications [16]. However, due to restrictions of injected doses of isotopes, the limited sensitivity (2 – 5 %), the high scatter fraction (40 – 50 %) and the resulting high signal to noise ratio requesting smoothing of data the principally possible spatial resolution can usually not be attained in PET studies.

Data Correction and Image Reconstruction

The unmatched capacity of PET is that images can be fully quantitative with a linear relationship between the tissue-concentration of the tracer and the measured counts. In order to utilise this quantifying power a number of corrections must be applied. The most important is attenuation correction caused by the tissue between annihilation event and detector, which can be measured by external positron-emitting sources rotating around the head or calculated from contours of the head and known attenuation coefficients of brain tissue and skull at 511 keV. The coincidence events detected in a PET camera are contaminated by accidental or random coincidences, when two unselected gamma rays activate detectors within the coincidence timing window, and scattered events, when one or both gamma rays are deviated on their way out of the head. Both errors can be measured and are corrected in the recorded data. Further corrections are necessary for different efficiency of the detectors and for count-rate dependent losses due to dead-time of detectors and electronics [17].

Image reconstruction converts the events detected by the PET scanner into tomographic images of the brain representing the distribution of the tracer. The images are reconstructed from the new data after the correction factors have been applied. Cross-calibration to a source of known concentration allows expressing regional radioactivity in absolute values. In small structures this quantitation is impaired by the partial volume effect due to the limitation in spatial resolution, which can be corrected by coregistration to MRI.

The data set for image reconstruction consists of the projection data for a detector ring as represented in a sinogram, a 2 D matric, where the vertical axis represents the angle of the projection line and the horizontal line represents the displacement of the projection line from the centre of the field of view. From this sinogram cross-sectional images are reconstructed using filtered backprojection [18] applying a spatially invariant filter to the projection data and distributing the counts from a sinogram element along the line in image space it represents. Filtered back projection can be modified for 3 D data sets [19]. In state-of-the-art high resolution scanners iterative methods are applied, which use maximation and minimation criteria to calculate images with the best matches for the measured projection data (Fourier rebinning-FORE-combined with ordered-subsets expectation-maximization – OSEM [20, 19, 21]), but require large computing power [22]).

Parameters for Activation Studies

Functional brain imaging is based on the relationship between changes in neuronal activity and changes in blood flow and metabolism of that region. Compared to other tissue, blood flow and metabolism of the brain, especially the gray matter is very high at rest and metabolic changes during activation are small and for cognitive tasks often less than 5 % of the control condition [23]. Whereas many studies demonstrated a linear relationship between neuronal activity and regional cerebral blood flow (rCBF) (e.g. [24, 25]), these changes in blood flow are not paralleled by appropriate increases in regional cerebral metabolic rate for oxygen ($rCMRO_2$) [26]). This discrepancy results in changes of the local concentration of oxygen in the microcirculation, giving rise to the BOLD (blood oxygen level dependent) signal [27] used in functional magnetic resonance imaging (fMRI). Changes in glucose utilization (CMRGlc) exceed the increase in oxygen consumption [26]. The increase of glycolysis during activation is not only due to the altered spiking activity of neurons, but also affected by synaptic activity as reflected by local field potentials [28]; for excitatory synaptic transmission this increased demand for glucose was attributed to stimulated metabolism of astrocytes necessary for clearance of glutamate from the synapse [29].

PET measures quantitatively rCBF and rCMRGl at rest and the changes due to functional activation, whereas fMRI observes relative changes in blood oxygenation levels. Regional changes of blood flow due to functional activity were measured with the 2 dimensional inert gas clearance methods using ^{199}Xe (review in [30]). With the introduction of PET it became possible to apply the quantitative autoradiographic deoxyglucose technique [8] to regional measurement of glucose metabolism using ^{18}Fluor-deoxyglucose (FDG) [31]. FDG is actively transported into the brain and metabolized by hexokinase to FDG-6-phosphat similarly to glucose. Further steps in the metabolic pathway are blocked by the ^{18}F labelling on position 2, and the rate of the transport and the first metabolic step can be described by a 3-compartment model consisting of plasma pool, FDG in tissue and FDG-6 ph concentration connected by kinetic constants for transport to and into vs out of the brain and phosphorylation / dephosphorylation of the compound. Quantitative determinations of rCMRGl require sequential brain scanning and arterial (or arterialised venous) blood sampling and therefore often relative regional changes of FDG uptake are used in functional activation studies. For reaching the balance between accumulation, trapping and clearing of nonmetabolized FDG 30 min are required, and usually 20 – 30 min are used for image acquisition. Therefore, repeat or rapid studies of functional states are not feasible, and due to the half-life of ^{18}F (110 min) resting and activation studies are usually performed on different days. With the FDG method the first functional studies were performed in the early 80s with visual stimulation [32].

The strategy to measure blood flow with PET adopted the autoradiographic technique [33]. This required the intravenous injection of a freely diffusible tracer, e.g. $H_2{}^{15}O$, and integration of the activity in the brain by PET over 1 min [34]. The short half-life of ^{15}O (123 sec) allows sufficient tracer to be administered to obtain good counting statistics within this short measuring times with acceptable radiation dose to the subject. Also, repeat measurements of blood flow can be performed every 10 – 15 min permitting follow-up of different activation states in one session. Quantification is straight forward since $H_2{}^{15}O$ accumulates in the brain in a linear fashion with respect to blood flow; usually arterial blood sampling is avoided and regional changes relative to whole brain activity are used for functional studies [35]. $H_2{}^{15}O$-PET assesses the signal from the brain tissue, whereas the BOLD signal for fMRI arises predominantly from blood in draining venules a few millimetres away from the tissue compartment in which neural activity takes place [36].

Performance and Analysis of Functional Studies

In brain activation studies rCBF or metabolism is measured during the performance of a task and the results are compared with control measurements in order to identify the brain regions involved in the task (Figure 1). The control state should include the same sensorimotor and cognitive activities as the task, except the specific process being investigated.

In studies of complex cognitive functions subjects may perform sequential tasks of increasing complexity; each experimental state is compared with the preceding one, so that successive differences reveal brain areas that were recruited serially.

For the determination of task related activation subtraction of the “at rest” image from the “task” image has been the preferential method in the beginning, when quantitative metabolic or flow images were used [32, 34]. In order to avoid arterial blood sampling, this approach was replaced by semiquantitative or relative procedures, in which control and task images are normalized to eliminate the effect of global fluctuations. Thus multiple studies can be compared by normalizing each separate study to the same total radioactivity in the brain [37]. A statistical test is then applied to the difference image to determine which changes are statistically significant.

Anatomical localization of task related changes can be obtained by stereotactic methods: For that purpose the line joining the anterior and posterior commissures of the brain (AP-PC line) is used as a reference for a common coordinate system in both, the PET and the images from a stereotactic brain atlas [38]. Additionally, PET images can be matched to MR images in individual subjects and these can be transformed onto a common anatomical brain representation [39].

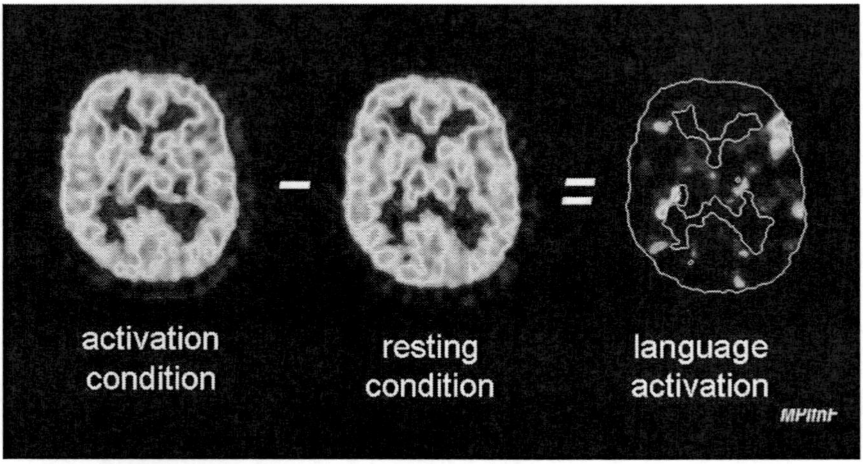

Figure 1. Localization of brain function by activation studies: the resting condition is subtracted from the activation condition.

For this purpose the images from different persons must be scaled to a common brain size, using linear or, to account for local variations in brain geometry, nonlinear scaling factors [40]. These complex procedures permit the identification of brain structures involved in various tasks, and form the basis for averaging responses in groups of patients, where summed subtraction images show an improved contrast of the local response. With the increased sensitivity of 3 D PET acquisition many runs with different tasks can be done in each individual with relatively low doses [10] which allow the examination of differences in information processing of different subjects, and permits longitudinal studies and investigation of patients with altered brain morphology.

Difference images are noisy and contain signals which might be relevant and irrelevant for the respective task performance. Therefore image analysis strategies are required to select the relevant information. One approach is to place regions of interest within the difference images to test specific hypotheses about areas affected by the specific task. This approach is based on the knowledge how the brain is organized and will miss additional relevant activation sites. It still has great value in the analysis of activation patterns in patients with brain lesions, e.g. strokes or tumors. An alternative approach more open to generating new hypotheses on localization of brain function is the determination of statistically significant responses regardless of their location or magnitude. With a voxel-based assessment PET activation studies were evaluated by change distribution analysis [41], which provided a mathematical proof for the subtraction paradigm. Most functional imaging studies are now analysed with some form of statistical parametric mapping, a procedure referring to the construction of spatially extended statistical processes to test a hypothesis about involvement of brain regions in particular functions [42]. Statistical parametric maps (SPMs) are images whose voxels are, under a null hypothesis, distributed according to a statistical probability density function [43]. Under the assumption of equivalence of activity (achieved by normalization of data) between resting and task related scans SPMs test defined null hypotheses and yield images of the significance of blood flow change. The simplest tests of significance are t-tests based on repeated measurements, but more sensitive and general approaches use analysis of variance (ANOVA) or analysis of covariance (ANCOVA), which removes the confounding effects of global CBF differences. The ANCOVA generates adjusted mean rCBF values for each experimental and control condition and an associated error variance at each voxel in the data set. These estimates are used to compute statistics for each voxel, and for each comparison of tasks or conditions of interest. This analytical procedure has a high power to identify specialized areas, and to demonstrate interactions among various regions in distributed systems by functional connectivity. Detailed descriptions of methodology, applications and results can be found in the extensive literature [44].

Limitations for PET Activation Studies

The serious limitation for PET activation studies is radiation exposure, which restricts the number of repeat studies especially in healthy volunteers despite 3D data acquisition and dose fractionation. The complexity of PET requiring a cyclotron for production of short lived isotopes and radio-chemistry for tracer preparation at the site of the scanner further impedes a broad application of this technology for cognitive studies. Therefore, PET activation studies were widely replaced by fMRI which is now the routine for multitask cognitive brain mapping. However, PET's role in this field is not only of historical interest, since it remains the gold standard for the quantification of physiological variables. PET can be used to investigate language production without articulation-related artifacts and – compared to MRI – is a relatively silent technique. It is also equally sensitive to signal throughout the brain, is not affected by inhomogeneities due to air-bone-tissue interfaces and does not – as echo-planar-imaging for fMRI – result in geometric distortion. The wider ring of PET scanners usually does not cause claustrophobia. Additionally, only PET permits to image changes in neurotransmitter and neuromodulator release and their involvement in the performance of complex cognitive tasks and behaviour [45] and the combination of activation studies with other interactions, e.g. transcranial magnetic stimulation [46].

FUNCTIONAL ACTIVATION IN HEALTHY SUBJECTS

Using radiotracer methods a tremendous number of functional studies were performed demonstrating activations in specific brain regions and inter-connected networks (reviews in [47, 48, 49]). In the following only a few examples can be given in which PET was leading for the analysis of functional activation patterns.

Visual System

The first functional mapping studies were performed in the visual system [32] in which increased regional metabolic rates for glucose were demonstrated in relation to intensity and complexity of the stimuli and involvement of visual association cortex was observed with complex interpretation. Topographic representation of different areas of the retina with presentation of central vision near the occipital pole could be shown [50]. In a complex analysis of varying successive visual stimuli Zeki et al (1991) [51] could localize the perception of motion on the convexity of the hemisphere at the junction of the temporal and occipital cortex and the perception of colour to the fusiform gyrus in the inferior part of the occipital gyrus. Matching of faces activated a region of the occipito-temporal cortex while spatial locations were represented in the lateral superior parietal cortex [52].

Auditory System

Activation of the temporal cortex occurs with a wide variety of auditory stimuli, but distinguishing between two tunes depended on the analysis strategy, where musically naive subjects had greater activation of the right fronto-temporal region and musically sophisticated subjects had greater activations of the left temporal cortex [53]. The characteristics of the auditory stimulus affected the rCBF response in the primary auditory cortex, more complex stimuli including syllables and phonetic discrimination tasks activated additional areas required for further processing, on the superior temporal gyrus bilaterally, the left Broca's area and a superior parietal area [54].

Motor and Somatosensory Activation

During motor tasks both the pre-central and post-central cortices are activated reflecting the sensory control of movements [55, 56], but also the premotor cortex is involved in simple and more complex movements of the contralateral arm. Additionally, cerebellar as well as basal ganglia activations are observed. During complex movements of the upper limbs, especially the fingers and the eyes, also activation of the supplementary motor area was detected [56]. More complex tasks – motor planning and learning – involved additional areas in the premotor and prefrontal cortex as well as the superior parietal association cortex [57].

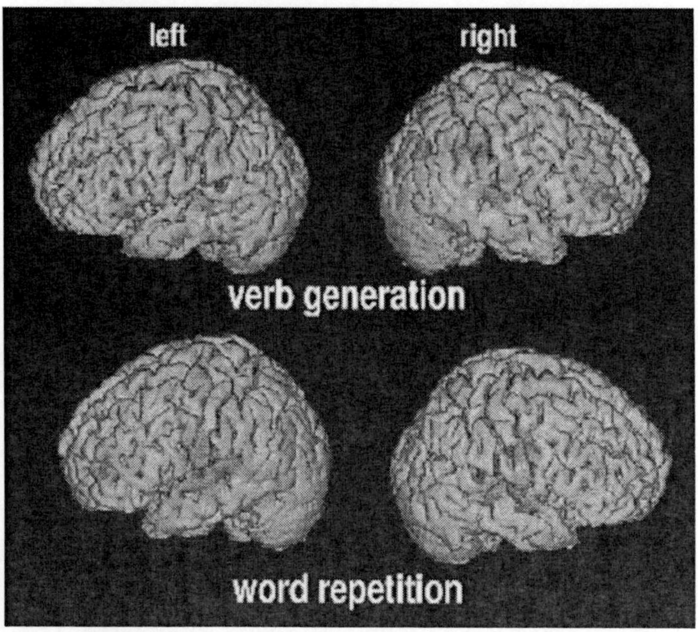

Figure 2. Cortical areas activated by verb generation and word repetition.

Responses to sensorimotor stimulation of the contralateral hand, face and foot correspond to the somatotopic organization of the primary sensory cortex [58], but also the supplementary motor area and the cerebellum receive sensory input. The response of the primary cortical area can be modulated by the attentive behaviour of the subject [59]. Brain processes involved in pain activate the thalamus and anterior cingulate, which is attributed to the emotional and attentional components of pain perception [60].

Language

PET studies were designed to investigate specific aspects of language processing and speech production. Processing of single words depended on the form of presentation (viewing or listening) and the type of response required (reading or repeating or generating verbs related to a noun). In successive tasks with increasing processing requirements Petersen et al [61] could demonstrate that visual presentation of words activated the primary and extrastriate occipital cortex, listening to words activated the superior temporal cortex bilaterally and the left temporoparietal cortex. Saying nouns activated the primary sensori-motor mouth area, supplementary motor area and left inferior frontal structures (Broca's area) (Figure. 2). The semantic task of generating an appropriate verb activated the left anterior prefrontal and cingulated cortex. Thus, different ways of stimulus presentation involved different primary and association areas, while output and semantic processing activated similar areas regardless of the type of stimulation. Based on additional studies with complex series of stimuli and processing tasks Price [62] has formulated a schematic model of language perception and speech production involving a complex connected network distributed over the whole brain. Further studies including repetitive transcranial magnetic simulation (rTMS) have revealed the influence of transcallosal inhibition for the development of left hemispheric dominance for speech and of the role of the left superior temporal gyrus (Wernicke region) for language interpretation [46, 63].

Cognition and Memory

PET activation studies have also been performed to study higher cortical functions, as attention, mental imagery and memory (review in [43, 47, 64, 65] but due to the complex design of these experiments and the necessity of multiple tasks requiring repeated injections of radioactive tracers they are the domain of fMRI.

However, PET has also pioneered this field with the first localization of attention to the cingulated cortex [66] and of memory functions to the dorsolateral frontal cortex [67, 68] and the hippocampus [69]. It must be stressed that PET permits to study the effects of various drugs on regional blood flow during memory-tasks, where the effect on serotoninergic nuclei (parahippocampal gyrus) and on dopaminergic areas (dorsolateral prefrontal cortex) could be visualized [70]. In recent experiments even the involvement of synaptic transmission, e.g. in the dopaminergic system, could be directly investigated [45].

ACTIVATION PATTERNS IN BRAIN DISEASE

Functional recovery after focal brain lesions is dependent on the adaptive plasticity of the cerebral cortex and of non-affected elements of the functional networks. After cortical injury the adjacent spared cortical tissue as well as more remote areas are altered resulting in changes in both excitatory and inhibitory neurotransmission involved in functional reorganization.

One consequence of cortical lesions is reduced collateral and transcallosal inhibition, which is expressed in activation of larger and even contralateral cortical areas during task performance, that are not involved in healthy volunteers. These activation patterns change in the course after a lesion and are related to recovery. Changes in activation patterns and their relationship to recovery were repeatedly studied after ischemic stroke.

Due to its outstanding significance for clinical rehabilitation the investigation of motor systems employing active motor tasks has been the focus of several functional imaging studies of post-stroke patients [71], reviews in [72, 73].

At the site of the injury, cortical responsiveness is reduced, but it increases over time related to the extent of recovery. The reorganisation of central nervous system elements is expressed in increased activity in brain regions distant from the lesion, in an increased activity in the contralateral hemisphere, and in somatotopic shifts within intact cortical regions.

How much functional neuroimaging can guide restorative interventions and yield insight into mechanisms of treatment effects is still a matter of debate [74].

POSTSTROKE APHASIA

Aphasia is a severely incapacitating symptom of stroke and is a main cause of functional disturbance. Estimates suggest that more than 20 % of patients suffering a stroke develop aphasia, 10 – 18 % of survivors are left with a persistent speech deficit [75]. Most patients with aphasia due to acute non-progressive brain damage, such as in the case of stroke or head injury, show some degree of recovery of language function during the days, months, or even years following the initial insult. The recuperation is variable, ranging from the hardly noticeable improvement of auditory comprehension of the global aphasia to the apparently complete recovery of the patient with mild fluent aphasia due to small subcortical stroke. It is also well known that improvement can be observed not only in patients submitted to language rehabilitation but also in cases that have not undergone any specific treatment.

Disturbance of Regional Metabolism and Flow versus Severity and Persistence of Language Deficit

Studies of glucose metabolism after stroke [76] have shown metabolic disturbances in the ipsilateral hemisphere caused by the lesion and contralateral hemisphere caused by functional deactivation (diaschisis) [77]. Most studies have been performed in right-handed individuals with language dominance in the left hemisphere. The left temporo-parietal region, in particular the angular gyrus, supramarginal gyrus, and lateral and transverse superior temporal gyrus are the most frequently and consistently impaired, and the degree of impairment is related to the severity of aphasia [78, 79]. In contrast, metabolic impairment in subcortical structures is related mainly to language fluency and other behavioural aspects, but not to aphasia severity [80]. In patients with aphasia attributable to purely subcortical strokes deactivation of temporo-parietal cortex is regularly found, which is probably responsible for the aphasic symptoms [81].

Recovery of metabolism in both hemispheres was correlated with recovery of aphasia. One specific region crucial for recovery of language perception has been found in the left temporo-parietal cortex [79, 82] and metabolic disturbance in these areas is related to outcome [83]. Investigations in the subacute state after stroke showed a highly significant correlation with language performance assessed at follow-up after 2 years [84]. The receptive language disorder correlated with rCMRGlc in the left temporal cortex and word fluency correlated with rCMRGlc in the left prefrontal cortex. These results indicate that the functional disturbance as measured by rCMRGlc in speech-relevant brain regions early after stroke is predictive of the eventual outcome of aphasia. However, not only functional deactivation (diaschisis) but also neuronal loss may contribute to metabolic and perfusional changes in the neighbourhood of the infarct, and the condition of the surrounding tissue may affect the recovery of individual patients. In this context it is important to note that early reperfusion to specific areas is able to restore disturbed function, as demonstrated for recovery of naming by reperfusion to the key areas BA37, BA 44/45 (Broca) and BA 22 (Wernicke) [85].

Changes in Activation Patterns versus Recovery of Language Function

On this basis it is not surprising that, in patients with a poor outcome of poststroke aphasia, metabolism in the hemisphere outside the infarct was significantly less than in those with good language recovery, indicating significant cell loss caused by the ischemic episode outside the ischemic core [86].

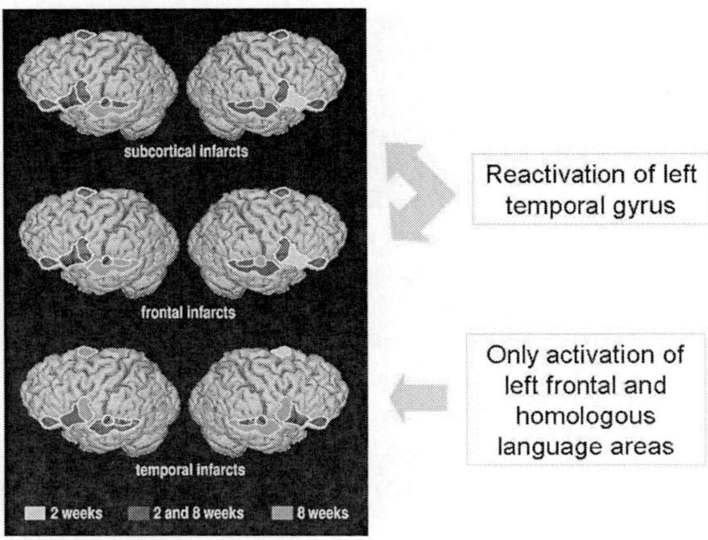

Figure 3. Activation patterns in patients with left hemispheric stroke 2 and 8 weeks after stroke. In the case of subcortical and frontal infarction, the left temporal areas are reactivated correlating to better recovery of language function. From Heiss et al 1999.

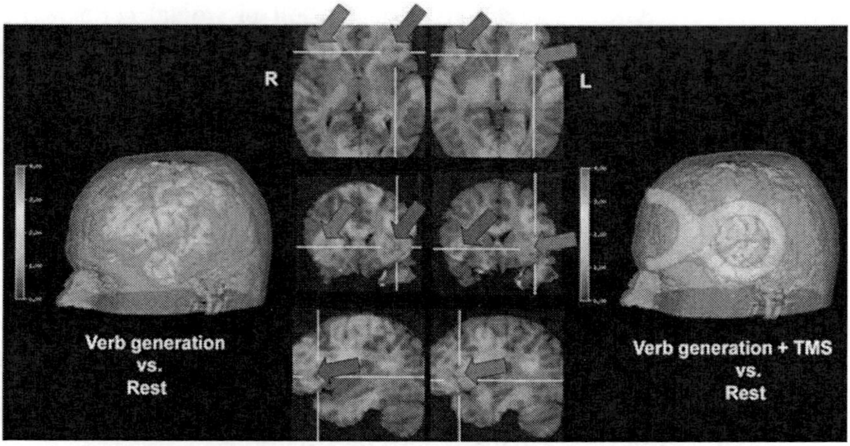

Figure 4. Effect of repetitive transcranial magnetic stimulation on activation pattern by verb generation. Activation pattern (A) and coil position (D) shown in 3 D rendering. Images in 3 dimensions (B) show activation of left inferior frontal gyrus during verb generation (red arrows), images (C) clearly show the decreased activation on the left (green arrow) and increased activity on the right side (red arrows) during rTMS interference. Modified from Thiel et al 2006.

In addition, the functionality of the network was reduced in patients with an eventual poor outcome; during task performance, patients with an eventual good recovery predominantly activated structures in the ipsilateral hemisphere. It must be kept in mind that aphasia symptoms – and consequently also activation patterns – improve with restoration of regional blood flow [87].

One of the central issues of aphasia research is the question why recovery from aphasia is taking place and what the responsible mechanisms for this recovery are. Converging evidence from clinical studies and neural imaging studies of aphasic patients suggest that primary candidates for recovery in right-handed, left-hemisphere language dominant patients include undamaged portions of the language network in the left hemisphere and – to a lesser extent – homologous right-hemisphere areas [88]. Since the language network is not confined to the dominant hemisphere, the role of the right hemisphere after infarcts in the left hemisphere has been addressed in several studies. Generally, more right hemispheric activations were seen in the subacute phase of an infarct with language activation than in normals with the same tasks [89-92]. Despite such responses in the right superior temporal gyrus especially in fluent Wernicke's patients [90, 93] and in the inferior frontal gyrus [89], efficient restoration of language is usually achieved only if left temporal areas are preserved and can be reintegrated into the functional network [94]. Only the basic function of mere word repetition appears to be sufficiently supported by sole right hemisphere activation [95]. Based on their study in chronic non-fluent aphasia patients Belin et al [96] suggested that the increased activation within the right hemisphere may be a marker of failed or faulty recovery attempts in the sense of maladaptive plasticity or the breakdown of normal interhemispheric control within the distributed neural network. Language recovery in the months immediately after aphasia onset was associated with regression of functional depression (diaschisis) in structurally unaffected regions, in particular in the right hemisphere [76, 92]. Right hemispheric activations after left frontal or temporal parietal damage are not related to the level of recovery [97] but may reflect transcallosal inhibition as a maladaptive neuronal reorganization rather than functional compensation [91]. Despite the brain recruits right hemispheric regions for speech processing when the left-hemispheric centres are impaired [98], outcome studies reveal that this strategy is significantly less effective than repair of the speech-relevant network in adults [99].

Changes in the activation pattern induced by repeating words in the course after ischemic stroke were related to recovery from poststroke aphasia [100]. Repeating words activated blood flow in 10 normal controls by more than 10 % relative to resting condition in both upper temporal gyri, by 5 – 10 % in planum temporale and Heschl gyrus of both sides and in the lower part of the central gyrus of the left side, and by less than 5 % in the left Broca area. This test procedure was applied to 23 patients with aphasia of different types. Morphological defects were defined on MRI/CT, and the patients were grouped according to the site of the lesion. Activation PET studies were performed in the subacute stage approximately 2 weeks after the stroke and repeated 6 weeks later. On matched MRIs regions of interest were defined in 14 identified structures of the bilateral language-related network.

The three groups of aphasic patients showed different patterns for activation in the acute and chronic phase, and their improvement was different: Whereas subcortical and frontal infarcts improved considerably in several tests, temporal infarcts showed only little improvement. These differences in improvement of speech deficits were reflected in different patterns of activation in the course after stroke (Figure 3): The subcortical and frontal groups improved substantially and activated the right inferior frontal gyrus and the right superior temporal gyrus (STG) at baseline and regained regional left STG activation at follow-up. The temporal group improved only in word comprehension; it activated the left Broca area and supplementary motor areas at baseline and the precentral gyrus bilaterally as well as the right STG at follow-up, but could not reactivate the left STG. Similar reactivation patterns were observed in smaller groups of patients [101, 102]. A recent study with repeated fMRI and parallel language testing from the acute to the chronic stage after stroke demonstrated a similar pattern [92]. All 14 patients recovered clinically as shown by a set of aphasia tests. In the acute phase (mean: 1.8 days post stroke) group analysis showed little early activation of non-infarcted left-hemispheric language structures, while in the subacute phase (12.1 days post stroke) a large increase of activation in the bilateral language network, with a peak in the right Broca-homologue occured. In the chronic phase (1321 days post stroke) a normalization of activation with re-shift to left-hemispheric areas was observed. This reorganization with recruitment of homologue language zones correlated with improvement, the normalization possibly reflected recovery and consolidation of the language system.

Effect of Treatment in Poststroke Aphasia

Whereas the effect of physiotherapy on improvement of sensorimotor deficits is unchallenged, the efficiency of speech therapy is still controversial, with several randomized controlled trials yielding no difference in outcome between treated and untreated groups [103, 104]. Many trials were undertaken to enhance the recovery from aphasia with adjuvant pharmacotherapy, but again, only a few studies demonstrated efficacy: In a double-blind placebo-controlled study Walker-Batson et al [105] described a significantly increased gain in score in patients treated with dextroamphetamine before speech therapy sessions compared to the placebo group, but the difference was not significant at 6 months follow-up. Similarly, donepezil improved the effect of speech therapy only temporarily [106]. A large Cochrane Review [107] identified piracetam as the only drug with a significant effect on recovery of language, which was also observed in a large multicentre trial [108]. The effect of piracetam is also reflected in altered activation patterns. In a placebo controlled double blind study [109] (2 x 2.4 g piracetam vs placebo) the piracetam group did significantly better especially in subtests reflecting the ability for spontaneous speech. These differences in improvement were also reflected in differences in the achieved activation patterns: In the piracetam group increase in activation was significantly higher in the left transverse temporal gyrus, the left triangular part of the inferior frontal gyrus, and the left posterior temporal gyrus after the treatment period compared with the initial measures. It might be concluded that piracetam as an adjuvant to speech therapy improves recovery of various language functions and that this effect is accompanied by task-related flow activation in eloquent areas of the left hemisphere. Other imaging studies with individualized aphasia treatment in small numbers of patients did not show conclusive changes in fMRI activation patterns (review in [110].

Combination of Repetitive Transcranial Magnetic Stimulation (rTMS) with Activated Imaging

rTMS is a non-invasive procedure to create electric currents in discrete brain areas [111] which depending on frequency, intensity, and duration can lead to transient increases and decreases in excitability of the affected cortex. Increases in relative cerebral blood volume in contralateral homologous language regions during overt propositional speech fMRI in chronic, non-fluent aphasia patients indicated over-activation of right language homologues [112]. This right hemisphere over-activation may represent a maladaptive strategy, as suggested previously by Belin et al [96] and Rosen et al [88] in their studies with chronic, non-fluent aphasia patients. This over-activation in the right homologous language areas can be interpreted as a result of decreased transcallosal inhibition due to damage of the specialized and lateralized speech areas [99].

Both types of inhibition – collateral ipsilateral and transcallosal contralateral – can be demonstrated by simultaneous rTMS and PET activation studies [46]. In six normal male volunteers the Broca area, as defined by maximal activation during verb generation in the left inferior frontal gyrus was stimulated by rTMS to interfere with normal language function. During verb generation, rCBF was decreased during rTMS ipsilateral under the coil, but increased ipsilateral outside the coil and in the contralateral homologous area (Figure 4). The effect of rTMS was accompanied by a prolongation of reaction time latencies to verbal stimuli.

The role of activation in the right hemisphere for residual language performance can be investigated by combining rTMS with functional imaging, e.g. PET [113]. Such an approach was used in 11 patients with predominantly non-fluent aphasia 2 weeks after left sided middle cerebral artery infarction [114]. rTMS stimulation sites were selected according to maximum flow activation within left and right inferior frontal gyrus (IFG). Of these patients three activated the left, eight the bilateral inferior frontal gyrus. rTMS (4 Hz for 20 sec.) resulted in increased reaction time latency or error rate in the word generation task in five patients with right IFG activation, indicating essential language function. In a verbal fluency task, these patients had a lower performance than patients with effects of rTMS only over the left IFG, suggesting a less effective compensatory potential of right sided network areas. These results were supported by studies in tumour patients [115], in which a significant correlation between the laterality index and the performance in a verbal fluency test was observed in the patients without right-positive TMS effect, whereas in patients with a predominant right-positive TMS effect the performance in the verbal fluency test was comparable with that in controls. This result may indicate that in a few patients with left hemispheric brain tumours the slow progression of damage leads to a shift in language function to the right hemisphere which can compensate for the defect on the left side.

Conclusion

The different dynamics of recovery of language function observed in patients after stroke and with tumours in the left hemisphere suggest various mechanisms for compensation of the lesion within the functional network. A hierarchy for effective recovery might be deduced from these data (Figure 4) [116]:

Best, even complete recovery of function can usually only be achieved by the restoration of the original activation pattern within the network of the dominant hemisphere; this is only feasible after small brain damage probably only affecting an area of minor importance permitting functional restitution of the main interconnected components.

If primary functional centres are damaged, reduction of collateral inhibition leads to activation of areas around the lesion; this intrahemispheric compensation involving secondary centres of the ipsilateral network is the basis for incomplete, but often satisfactory improvement of language function.

If ipsilateral network components are severely damaged, reduction of transcallosal inhibition causes activation of contralateral homotopic areas; this interhemispheric compensation involving homotopic contralesional areas contributes to some improvement in function, which is dependent on the extent of the functional shift between the hemispheres, but usually is not as efficient as intrahemispheric compensation. However, in some patients with slowly developing brain damage – and perhaps also an a priori not highly lateralized functional network – the language function can be completely shifted to the right hemisphere, and in these cases speech performance can be preserved or completely recover despite the damage in the left (previously dominant) hemisphere.

It must be shown in larger controlled trials if the blockade of inhibitory interaction by contralateral intact areas with rTMS [117] "increases the ability of the brain to undergo compensatory changes that improve behaviours" [118] and is an effective strategy to improve recovery of language function.

REFERENCES

[1] Ter-Pogossian MM, Eichling JO, Davis DO, Welch MJ, Metzger JM. The determination of regional cerebral blood flow by means of water labeled with radioactive oxygen 15. *Radiology*. 1969;93:31-40.

[2] Ter-Pogossian MM, Eichling JO, Davis DO, Welch MJ. The measure in vivo of regional cerebral oxygen utilization by means of oxyhemoglobin labeled with radioactive oxygen - 15. *Journal of Clinical Investigation*. 1970;49:381-391.

[3] Cormack AM. Reconstruction of densities from their projections, with applications in radiological physics. *Phys. Med. Biol.* 1973;18:195-207.

[4] Phelps ME, Hoffman EJ, Mullemi NA, Ter-Pogossian MM. Application of annihilation coincidence detection to transaxial reconstruction tomography. *J. Nucl. Med.* 1975;16:210-224.

[5] Ter-Pogossian MM, Phelps ME, Hoffman EJ, Mullani NA. A positron emission transaxial tomograph for nuclear imaging (pett). *Radiology*. 1975;114:89-98.

[6] Phelps ME, Hoffman EJ, Huang SC, Kuhl DE. Ecat: A new computerized tomographic imaging system for positron-emitting radiopharmaceuticals. *J. Nucl. Med.* 1978;19:635-647.

[7] Sakurada O, Kennedy C, Jehle J, Brown JD, Carbin GL, Sokoloff L. Measurement of local cerebral blood flow with iodo(14 c)antipyrine. *Am. J. Physiol.* 1978;234:H59-H66.

[8] Sokoloff L, Reivich M, Kennedy C, Des Rosiers MH, Patlak CS, Pettigrew KD, Sakurada O, Shinohara M. The (14 c)-deoxyglucose method for the measurement of local cerebral glucose utilization: Theory, procedure, and normal values in the conscious and anesthetized albino rat. *J. Neurochem.* 1977;28:897-916.

[9] Ter-Pogossian MM. The origins of positron emission tomography. *Semin. Nucl. Med.* 1992;22:140-149.

[10] Cherry SR, Phelps ME. Imaging brain function with positron emission tomography. In: Toga AW, Mazziotta JC, eds. *Brain mapping: The methods*. San Diego: Academic Press; 1996.

[11] Eriksson L, Bohm C, Kesselberg M, Blomqvist G, Litton J, Widen L, Bergström M, Ericson K, Greitz T. A four ring positron camera system for emission tomography of the brain. *IEEE Transactions on Nuclear Science*. 1982;29:539-543.

[12] Casey ME, Nutt R. A multicrystal two dimensional bgo detector system for positron emission tomography. *IEEE Trans. Nucl. Sci.* 1986;NS-33:460-463.

[13] Wienhard K, Dahlbom M, Eriksson L, Michel C, Bruckbauer T, Pietrzyk U, Heiss WD. The ecat exact hr: Performance of a new high resolution positron scanner. *J. Comput. Assist. Tomogr*. 1994;18:110-118.

[14] Wienhard K, Schmand M, Casey ME, Baker K, Bao J, Eriksson L, Jones WF, Knoess C, Lenox M, Lercher M, Luk P, Michel C, Reed JH, Richerzhagen N, Treffert J, Vollmar S, Young JW, Heiss WD, Nutt R. The ecat hrrt: Performance and first clinical application of the new high resolution research tomograph. *IEEE Transactions on Nuclear Science*. 2002;49:104-110.

[15] Cherry SR, Shao Y, Silverman RW, Meadors K, Siegel S, Chatziioannou A, Young JW, Jones WF, Moyers JC, Newport D, Boutefnouchet A, Farquhar TH, Andreaco M, Paulus MJ, Binkley DM, Nutt R, Phelps ME. Micropet: A high-resolution pet scanner for imaging small animals. *IEEE Transactions on Nuclear Science*. 1997;44:1161-1166.

[16] de Jong HWAM, van Velden FHP, Kloet RW, Buijs FL, Boellaard R, Lammertsma AA. Performance evaluation of the ecat hrrt: An lso-lyso double layer high resolution, high sensitivity scanner. *Phys. Med. Biol.* 2007;52:1505-1526.

[17] Hoffmann EJ, Guerrero TM, Germano G, al. e. Pet system calibration and corrections for quantitative and spatially accurate images. *IEEE Trans Nucl. Sci.* 1989;NS-36:1108-1112.

[18] Brooks RA, Di Chiro G. Principles of computer assisted tomography (cat) in radiographic and radioisotopic imaging. *Phys. Med. Biol.* 1976;21:689-732.

[19] Defrise M, Kinahan PE, Townsend DW, Michel C, Sibomana M, Newport D. Exact and approximate rebinning algorithms for 3-d pet data. *IEEE Trans. Med. Imag*. 1997;16:145-158.

[20] Hudson HM, Larkin RS. Accelerated image reconstruction using ordered subsets of projection data. *IEEE Transactions on Medical Imaging*. 1994;13:68-78.

[21] Liu X, Comtat C, Michel C, Kinahan P, Defrise M, Townsend D. Comparison of 3-d reconstruction with 3x-osem and with fore + osem for pet. *IEEE Transactions on Medical Imaging*. 2001;20:804-814.

[22] Vollmar S, Michel C, Treffert JT, Newport DF, Casey M, Knoess C, Wienhard K, Liu X, Defrise M, Heiss WD. Heinzelcluster: Accelerated reconstruction for fore and osem3d. *Physics in Medicine and Biology*. 2002;47 2651-2658.

[23] Clarke DD, Sokoloff L. Circulation and energy metabolism of the brain. In: Siegel G, Agranoff B, Albers RW, Fisher S, eds. *Basic neurochemistry: Molecular, cellular, and medical aspects, 6th ed.* Philadelphia: Lippincott-Raven; 1999:637-669.

[24] Heiss WD, Turnheim M, Vollmer R, Rappelsberger P. Coupling between neuronal activity and focal blood flow in experimental seizures. *ElectroencephclinNeurophysiol*. 1979;47:396-403.

[25] Raichle ME. A brief history of human functional brain mapping. In: Toga AW, Mazziotta JC, eds. *Brain mapping: The systems*. San Diego: Academic Press; 2000:33-75.

[26] Fox PT, Raichle ME, Mintun MA, Dence C. Nonoxidative glucose consumption during focal physiologic neural activity. *Science*. 1988;241:462-464.

[27] Ogawa S, Lee TM, Kay AR, Tank DW. Brain magnetic resonance imaging with contrast dependent on blood oxygenation. *Proc. Natl. Acad. Sci. U S A*. 1990;87:9868-9872.

[28] Sharp FR. Relative cerebral glucose uptake of neuronal perikarya and neuropil determined with 2-deoxyglucose in resting and swimming rat. *Brain Res*. 1976;110:127-139.

[29] Magistretti PJ, Pellerin L. Cellular bases of brain energy metabolism and their relevance to functional brain imaging: Evidence for a prominent role of astrocytes. *Cereb. Cortex*. 1996;6:50-61.

[30] Lassen NA, Ingvar DH, Skinhoj E. Brain function and blood flow. *Sci. Am*. 1978;239:62-71.

[31] Reivich M, Kuhl D, Wolf A, Greenberg J, Phelps M, Ido T, Casella V, Fowler J, Hoffman E, Alavi A, Som P, Sokoloff L. The (18 f)fluorodeoxyglucose method for the measurement of local cerebral glucose utilization in man. *Circulation Research*. 1979;44:127-137.

[32] Phelps ME, Kuhl DE, Mazziotta JC. Metabolic mapping of brain's response to visual stimulation: Studies in humans. *Science.* 1981;211:1445-1448.

[33] Landau WM, Freygang WH, Jr., Roland LP, Sokoloff L, Kety SS. The local circulation of the living brain; values in the unanesthetized and anesthetized cat. *Trans. Am. Neurol. Assoc.* 1955;80:125-129.

[34] Herscovitch P, Markham J, Raichle ME. Brain blood flow measured with intravenous h 2 15 o. I. Theory and error analysis. *J. Nucl. Med.* 1983;24:782-789.

[35] Fox PT, Mintun MA, Raichle ME, Herscovitch P. A noninvasive approach to quantitative functional brain mapping with h 2 15 o and positron emission tomography. *J. Cereb. Blood Flow Metab.* 1984;4:329-333.

[36] Ugurbil K, Toth L, Kim DS. How accurate is magnetic resonance imaging of brain function? *Trends Neurosci.* 2003;26:108-114.

[37] Mazziotta JC, Huang SC, Phelps ME, Carson RE, MacDonald NS, Mahoney K. A noninvasive positron computed tomography technique using oxygen-15-labeled-water for the evaluation of neurobehavioral task batteries. *J. Cereb. Blood Flow Metab.* 1985;5:70-78.

[38] Talairach J, Tournoux P. *Co-planar stereotaxic atlas of the human brain.* New York: Thieme; 1988.

[39] Seitz RJ, Bohm C, Greitz T, Roland PE, Eriksson L, Blomqvist G, Rosenqvist G, Nordell B. Accuracy and precision of the computerized brain atlas program for localization and quantification in positron emission tomography. *J. Cereb. Blood Flow Metab.* 1990;10:443-457.

[40] Friston KJ, Frith CD, Liddle PF, Frackowiak RS. Plastic transformation of pet images. *J. Comput. Assist. Tomogr.* 1991;15:634-639.

[41] Fox PT, Mintun MA. Noninvasive functional brain mapping by change-distribution analysis of averaged pet images of h215o tissue activity. *J. Nucl. Med.* 1989;30:141-149.

[42] Friston KJ, Frith CD, Liddle PF, Frackowiak RS. Comparing functional (pet) images: The assessment of significant change. *J. Cereb. Blood Flow Metab.* 1991;11:690-699.

[43] Frackowiak RSJ, Friston KJ. Functional neuroanatomy of the human brain: Positron emission tomography - a new neuroanatomical technique. *J. Anatomy.* 1994;184:211-225.

[44] Friston K, Ashburner J, Kiebel S. *Statistical parametric mapping: The analysis of functional brain images.* Oxford: Elsevier Science and Technology Books; 2007.

[45] Koepp MJ, Gunn RN, Lawrence AD, Cunningham VJ, Dagher A, Jones T, Brooks DJ, Bench CJ, Grasby PM. Evidence for striatal dopamine release during a video game. *Nature*. 1998;393:266-268.

[46] Thiel A, Schumacher B, Wienhard K, Gairing S, Kracht LW, Wagner R, Haupt WF, Heiss WD. Direct demonstration of transcallosal disinhibition in language networks. *J. Cereb. Blood Flow Metab.* 2006;26:1122-1127.

[47] Herscovitch P. Functional mapping of the human brain. In: Wayner HNJ, Szabo S, Buchanan JW, eds. *Principles of nuclear medicine* Philadelphia: W. B. Saunders 1995:514-531.

[48] Bigler ED, Turkheimer E. *Neuropsychological function and brain imaging*. New York: Plenum; 1989.

[49] Phelps ME. Pet: A biological imaging technique. *Neuro. Chem. Res.* 1991;16:929-940.

[50] Fox PT, Miezin FM, Allman JM, Van Essen DC, Raichle ME. Retinotopic organization of human visual cortex mapped with positron-emission tomography. *J. Neurosci.* 1987;7:913-922.

[51] Zeki S, Watson JDG, Lueck CJ, Friston KJ, Kennard C, Frackowiak RSJ. A direct demonstration of functional specialization in human visual cortex. *J. Neurosci.* 1991;11:641-649.

[52] Haxby JV, Grady CL, Horwitz B, Ungerleider LG, Mishkin M, Carson RE, Herscovitch P, Schapiro MB, Rapoport SI. Dissociation of object and spatial visual processing pathways in human extrastriate cortex. *Proc. Natl. Acad. Sci. USA*. 1991;88:1621-1625.

[53] Mazziotta JC, Phelps ME, Carson RE, Kuhl DE. Tomographic mapping of human cerebral metabolism: Auditory stimulation. *Neurology*. 1982;32:921-937.

[54] Zatorre RJ, Evans AC, Meyer E, Gjedde A. Lateralization of phonetic and pitch discrimination in speech processing. *Science*. 1992;256:846-849.

[55] Grafton ST, Woods RP, Mazziotta JC, Phelps ME. Somatotopic mapping of the primary motor cortex in humans: Activation studies with cerebral blood flow and positron emission tomography. *J. Neurophysiol.* 1991;66:735-743.

[56] Colebatch JG, Deiber MP, Passingham RE, Friston KJ, Frackowiak RSJ. Regional cerebral blood flow during voluntary arm and hand movements in human subjects. *Journal of Neurophysiology*. 1991;65:1392-1401.

[57] Seitz RJ, Roland PE. Learning of sequential finger movements in man: A combined kinematic and positron emission tomography (pet) study. *Eur. J. Neurosci.* 1992;4:154-165.

[58] Fox PT, Burton H, Raichle ME. Mapping human somatosensory cortex with positron emission tomography. *J. Neurosurg.* 1987;67:34-43.

[59] Meyer E, Ferguson SSG, Zatorre RJ, Alivisatos B, Marrett S, Evans AC, Hakim AM. Attention modulates somatosensory cerebral blood flow response to vibrotactile stimulation as measured by positron emission tomography. *Ann. Neurol.* 1991;29:440-443.

[60] Duncan GH, Bushnell MC, Talbot JD, Evans AC, Meyer E, Marrett S. Localization of responses to pain (letter). *Science.* 1992a;255:215 – 216.

[61] Petersen SE, Fox PT, Posner MI, Mintun M, Raichle ME. Positron emission tomographic studies of the cortical anatomy of single-word processing. *Nature.* 1988;331:585-589.

[62] Price CJ. The anatomy of language: Contributions from functional neuroimaging. *Journal of Anatomy.* 2000;197 Pt 3:335-359.

[63] Karbe H, Herholz K, Halber M, Heiss WD. Collateral inhibition of transcallosal activity facilitates functional brain asymmetry. *J. Cereb. Blood Flow Metab.* 1998;18:1157-1161.

[64] Cabeza R, Kingstone A. *Handbook of functional neuroimaging of cognition.* London: The MIT Press; 2006.

[65] Law I. Human brain mapping under increasing cognitive complexity using regional cerebral blood flow measurements and positron emission tomography. *Dan. Med. Bull.* 2007;54:289-305.

[66] Pardo JV, Pardo PJ, Janer KW, Raichle ME. The anterior cingulate cortex mediates processing selection in the stroop attentional conflict paradigm. *Proc. Natl. Acad. Sci. U S A.* 1990;87:256-259.

[67] Petrides M, Alivisatos B, Meyer E, Evans AC. Functional activation of the human frontal cortex during the performance of verbal working memory tasks. *Proc. Natl. Acad. Sci. U S A.* 1993;90:878-882.

[68] Courtney SM, Ungerleider LG, Keil K, Haxby JV. Object and spatial visual working memory activate separate neural systems in human cortex. *Cereb. Cortex.* 1996;6:39-49.

[69] Squire LR, Ojemann JG, Miezin FM, Petersen SE, Videen TO, Raichle ME. Activation of the hippocampus in normal humans: A functional anatomical study of memory. *Proc. Natl. Acad. Sci. USA.* 1992;89:1837-1841.

[70] Grasby PM, Friston KJ, Bench CJ, Frith CD, Paulesu E, Cowen PJ, Liddle PF, Frackowiak RS, Dolan R. The effect of apomorphine and

buspirone on regional cerebral blood flow during the performance of a cognitive task-measuring neuromodulatory effects of psychotropic drugs in man. *Eur. J. Neurosci.* 1992;4:1203-1212.

[71] Chollet F, Di Piero V, Wise RJS, Brooks DJ, Dolan RJ, Frackowiak RSJ. The functional anatomy of motor recovery after stroke in humans: A study with positron emission tomography. *Ann. Neurol.* 1991;29:63-71.

[72] Weiller C. Imaging recovery from stroke. *Exp. Brain Res.* 1998;123:13-17.

[73] Cramer SC. Repairing the human brain after stroke: I. Mechanisms of spontaneous recovery. *Ann. Neurol.* 2008;63:272-287.

[74] Cramer SC. Repairing the human brain after stroke. Ii. Restorative therapies. *Ann. Neurol.* 2008;63:549-560.

[75] Wade DT, Hewer RL, David RM, Enderby PM. Aphasia after stroke: Natural history and associated deficits. *J. Neurol. Neurosurg. Psychiatry.* 1986;49:11-16.

[76] Cappa SF, Perani D, Grassi F, Bressi S, Alberoni M, Franceschi M, Bettinardi V, Todde S, Fazio F. A pet follow-up study of recovery after stroke in acute aphasics. *Brain Lang.* 1997;56:55-67.

[77] Feeney DM, Baron JC. Diaschisis. *Stroke.* 1986;17:817-830.

[78] Metter EJ, Hanson WR, Jackson CA, Kempler D, Van Lancker D, Mazziotta JC, Phelps ME. Temporoparietal cortex in aphasia. Evidence from positron emission tomography. *Arch. Neurol.* 1990;47:1235-1238.

[79] Karbe H, Herholz K, Szelies B, Pawlik G, Wienhard K, Heiss WD. Regional metabolic correlates of token test results in cortical and subcortical left hemispheric infarction. *Neurology.* 1989;39:1083-1088.

[80] Metter EJ, Riege WH, Hanson WR, Jackson CA, Kempler D, Van Lancker D. Subcortical structures in aphasia. An analysis based on (18 f)-fluorodeoxyglucose, positron emission tomography, and computed tomography. *Arch. Neurol.* 1988;45:1229-1234.

[81] Kumar R, Masih AK, Pardo J. Global aphasia due to thalamic hemorrhage: A case report and review of the literature. *Arch. Phys. Med. Rehabil.* 1996;77:1312-1315.

[82] Metter EJ, Kempler D, Jackson CA, Hanson WR, Riege WH, Camras LR, Mazziotta JC, Phelps ME. Cerebellar glucose metabolism in chronic aphasia. *Neurology.* 1987;37:1599-1606.

[83] Heiss WD, Emunds HG, Herholz K. Cerebral glucose metabolism as a predictor of rehabilitation after ischemic stroke. *Stroke.* 1993;24:1784-1788.

[84] Karbe H, Kessler J, Herholz K, Fink GR, Heiss WD. Long-term prognosis of poststroke aphasia studied with positron emission tomography. *Arch. Neurol.* 1995;52:186-190.

[85] Hillis AE, Kleinman JT, Newhart M, Heidler-Gary J, Gottesman R, Barker PB, Aldrich E, Llinas R, Wityk R, Chaudhry P. Restoring cerebral blood flow reveals neural regions critical for naming. *J. Neurosci.* 2006;26:8069-8073.

[86] Heiss WD, Kessler J, Karbe H, Fink GR, Pawlik G. Cerebral glucose metabolism as a predictor of recovery from aphasia in ischemic stroke. *Arch. Neurol.* 1993;50:958-964.

[87] Jordan LC, Hillis AE. Disorders of speech and language: Aphasia, apraxia and dysarthria. *Curr. Opin. Neurol.* 2006;19:580-585.

[88] Rosen HJ, Petersen SE, Linenweber MR, Snyder AZ, White DA, Chapman L, Dromerick AW, Fiez JA, Corbetta MD. Neural correlates of recovery from aphasia after damage to left inferior frontal cortex. *Neurology.* 2000;55 1883-1894.

[89] Ohyama M, Senda M, Kitamura S, Ishii K, Mishina M, Terashi A. Role of the nondominant hemisphere and undamaged area during word repetition in poststroke aphasics - a pet activation study. *Stroke.* 1996;27:897-903.

[90] Weiller C, Isensee C, Rijntjes M, Huber W, Müller S, Bier D, Dutschka K, Woods RP, Noth J, Diener HC. Recovery from wernicke's aphasia: A positron emission tomographic study. *Ann. Neurol.* 1995;37:723-732.

[91] Price CJ, Crinion J. The latest on functional imaging studies of aphasic stroke. *Curr. Opin. Neurol.* 2005;18:429-434.

[92] Saur D, Lange R, Baumgaertner A, Schraknepper V, Willmes K, Rijntjes M, Weiller C. Dynamics of language reorganization after stroke. *Brain.* 2006;129:1371-1384.

[93] Musso M, Weiller C, Kiebel S, Müller SP, Bülau P, Rijntjes M. Training-induced brain plasticity in aphasia. *Brain.* 1999;122 1781-1790.

[94] Gainotti G. The riddle of the right hemisphere's contribution to the recovery of language. *Eur. J. Disord. Commun.* 1993;28:227-246.

[95] Berthier ML, Starkstein SE, Leiguarda R, Ruiz A, Mayberg HS, Wagner H, Price TR, Robinson RG. Transcortical aphasia. Importance of the nonspeech dominant hemisphere in language repetition. *Brain.* 1991;114 (Pt 3):1409-1427.

[96] Belin P, van Eeckhout P, Zilbovicius M, Remy P, Francois C, Guillaume S, Chain F, Rancurel G, Samson Y. Recovery from nonfluent aphasia

after melodic intonation therapy: A pet study. *Neurology*. 1996;47:1504-1511.

[97] Fernandez B, Cardebat D, Demonet JF, Joseph PA, Mazaux JM, Barat M, Allard M. Functional mri follow-up study of language processes in healthy subjects and during recovery in a case of aphasia. *Stroke*. 2004;35:2171-2176.

[98] Raboyeau G, De Boissezon X, Marie N, Balduyck S, Puel M, Bezy C, Demonet JF, Cardebat D. Right hemisphere activation in recovery from aphasia: Lesion effect or function recruitment? *Neurology*. 2008;70:290-298.

[99] Karbe H, Thiel A, Weber-Luxenburger G, Herholz K, Kessler J, Heiss WD. Brain plasticity in poststroke aphasia: What is the contribution of the right hemisphere? *Brain Lang*. 1998;64:215-230.

[100] Heiss WD, Kessler J, Thiel A, Ghaemi M, Karbe H. Differential capacity of left and right hemispheric areas for compensation of poststroke aphasia. *AnnNeurol*. 1999;45:430-438.

[101] Cao Y, Vikingstad EM, George KP, Johnson AF, Welch KMA. Cortical language activation in stroke patients recovering from aphasia with functional mri. *Stroke*. 1999;30:2331-2340.

[102] Warburton E, Price CJ, Swinburn K, Wise RJS. Mechanisms of recovery from aphasia: Evidence from positron emission tomography studies. *JNeurolNeurosurgPsychiatry*. 1999;66:155-161.

[103] Greener J, Enderby P, Whurr R. Speech and language therapy for aphasia following stroke (cochrane review). *The Cochrane Library 3*. 2001;Oxford: Update Software.

[104] Ferro JM, Mariano G, Madureira S. Recovery from aphasia and neglect. *CerebrovascDis*. 1999;9 (Suppl. 5):6-22.

[105] Walker-Batson D, Curtis S, Natarajan R, Ford J, Dronkers N, Salmeron E, Lai J, Unwin DH. A double-blind, placebo-controlled study of the use of amphetamine in the treatment of aphasia. *Stroke*. 2001;32:2093-2098.

[106] Berthier ML, Green C, Higueras C, Fernandez I, Hinojosa J, Martin MC. A randomized, placebo-controlled study of donepezil in poststroke aphasia. *Neurology*. 2006;67:1687-1689.

[107] Greener J, Enderby P, Whurr R. Pharmacological treatment for aphasia following stroke (protocol for a cochrane review). *The Cochrane Library 3*. 2001;Oxford: Update Software Orgogozo JM. Piracetam in the treatment of acute stroke. *Cns Drugs*. 1998;9:41-49.

[108] Kessler J, Thiel A, Karbe H, Heiss WD. Piracetam improves activated blood flow and facilitates rehabilitation of poststroke aphasic patients. *Stroke*. 2000;31:2112-2116.

[109] Crinion JT, Leff AP. Recovery and treatment of aphasia after stroke: Functional imaging studies. *Curr. Opin. Neurol.* 2007;20:667-673.

[110] Pascual-Leone A, Davey N, Wassermann EM, Rothwell J, Puri B. *Handbook of transcranial magnetic stimulation*. London: Arnold Press; 2002.

[111] Naeser MA, Martin PI, Baker EH, Hodge SM, Sczerzenie SE, Nicholas M, Palumbo CL, Goodglass H, Wingfield A, Samaraweera R, Harris G, Baird A, Renshaw P, Yurgelun-Todd D. Overt propositional speech in chronic nonfluent aphasia studied with the dynamic susceptibility contrast fmri method. *Neuroimage*. 2004;22:29-41.

[112] Siebner HR, Takano B, Peinemann A, Schwaiger M, Conrad B, Drzezga A. Continuous transcranial magnetic stimulation during positron emission tomography: A suitable tool for imaging regional excitability of the human cortex. *Neuroimage*. 2001;14:883-890.

[113] Winhuisen L, Thiel A, Schumacher B, Kessler J, Rudolf J, Haupt WF, Heiss WD. Role of the contralateral inferior frontal gyrus in recovery of language function in poststroke aphasia: A combined repetitive transcranial magnetic stimulation and positron emission tomography study. *Stroke*. 2005;36:1759-1763.

[114] Thiel A, Habedank B, Herholz K, Kessler J, Winhuisen L, Haupt WF, Heiss WD. From the left to the right: How the brain compensates progressive loss of language function. *Brain Lang*. 2006;98:57-65.

[115] Heiss WD, Thiel A. A proposed regional hierarchy in recovery of post-stroke aphasia. *Brain Lang*. 2006;98:118-123.

[116] Naeser MA, Martin PI, Nicholas M, Baker EH, Seekins H, Kobayashi M, Theoret H, Fregni F, Maria-Tormos J, Kurland J, Doron KW, Pascual-Leone A. Improved picture naming in chronic aphasia after tms to part of right broca's area: An open-protocol study. *Brain Lang*. 2005;93:95-105.

[117] Ridding MC, Rothwell JC. Therapeutic use of rtms. *Nat. Rev. Neurosci.* 2007;8:559-567.

In: Medical Imaging
Editors: M. D'Elia and A. Madaffari
ISBN: 978-1-62081-049-1

Chapter 7

REAL-TIME FUNCTIONAL MAGNETIC RESONANCE IMAGING AND ITS APPLICATIONS

Shaolin Yang, Thomas J. Ross and Yihong Yang
Neuroimaging Research Branch, National Institute on Drug Abuse
Baltimore, MD, US

ABSTRACT

Functional magnetic resonance imaging (fMRI) is a noninvasive imaging technique that is able to detect hemodynamic changes associated with neuronal activity in vivo. In the past decade, it has been used extensively for mapping functional neuroanatomy in basic neuroscience and clinical applications. A typical fMRI study includes acquisition of a time series of images (during which the subject is instructed to perform certain tasks) and offline processing and analysis of the image series. In real-time fMRI (rtfMRI), however, image processing and analysis start shortly after the beginning of the scan and then follow the image acquisition procedure as closely as possible. Real-time fMRI provides not only a useful tool for effective quality assurance of fMRI studies, but also opportunities for designing functional examinations with interactive controls and feedback.

In this chapter, we describe the basic concept and technical solution of rtfMRI, with a focus on a technique that we have recently developed and implemented on a Siemens 3T MRI scanner. We then demonstrate potential applications of rtfMRI techniques for neurofeedback and motion artifact reduction. In particular, we present a novel method of voluntary head-motion suppression using the feedback of the subject's own motion information in real time. This method was tested and the possible influence on the performance of tasks in fMRI study was assessed utilizing a commonly used working memory task. Our experiments showed that significant suppression of head motion was achieved consistently while the influence on the performance of task and the interference to brain activation could be minimized by careful design of the feedback system.

Keywords: functional magnetic resonance imaging (fMRI), real-time fMRI (rtfMRI), neurofeedback, head motion, BOLD

INTRODUCTION

In the last decade, we have experienced a renaissance in neuroimaging with the emergence of functional Magnetic Resonance Imaging (fMRI). FMRI is a noninvasive imaging technique that is able to detect hemodynamic changes putatively associated with neuronal activity *in vivo*. The origins of this renaissance can be traced to a convergence of discoveries and technologies. Ogawa's discovery of the Blood Oxygen Level Dependant (BOLD) effect that documented changes in concentration of paramagnetic deoxyhemoglobin lead to changes in local magnetic field inhomogeneity and hence changes in the MRI signal [1,2]. The BOLD effect is consistent with an early discovery by Fox et al. [3] that reported a regional overperfusion in response to neuronal activation obtained from positron emission tomography. The availability of single-shot MRI imaging techniques such as echo planar imaging [4] and spiral imaging [5] made it possible to image the entire brain, at spatial resolution of the order of millimeters, in seconds. So we are now able to image in seconds changes in blood deoxyhemoglobin as a result of perfusion changes related to neuronal activation – BOLD fMRI.

FMRI based on the BOLD effect has become the cornerstone of neuroimaging research. In the past decade, it has been used extensively for mapping functional neuroanatomy in basic neuroscience and clinical applications. There are a number of steps to be performed between data acquisition and the final statistical map. These can include reconstruction of the thousands to tens of thousands of slices, motion correction, spatial normalization, spatial filtering, temporal filtering and modeling of the time-course data.

Many of these steps are computationally intensive. However, Moore's law, the observation that number transistors – and hence computing power – doubles roughly every 18 months, has continued unabated [6] such that tasks like reconstruction that used to require expensive array processors are now done with desktop personal computers. Additionally, it has become relatively easy to combine PCs into a parallel processing cluster for greater performance [7]. By simplifying some of the processing steps, it is now possible to perform fMRI analysis in "real time."

What is meant by real-time fMRI (rtfMRI)? Clearly, despite computational improvements, the above steps take an appreciable amount of time. "Real-time" is typically defined as taking less time than other relevant time scales. For fMRI, the relevant time scale is the repetition time (TR), the time required to acquire one complete set of slices.

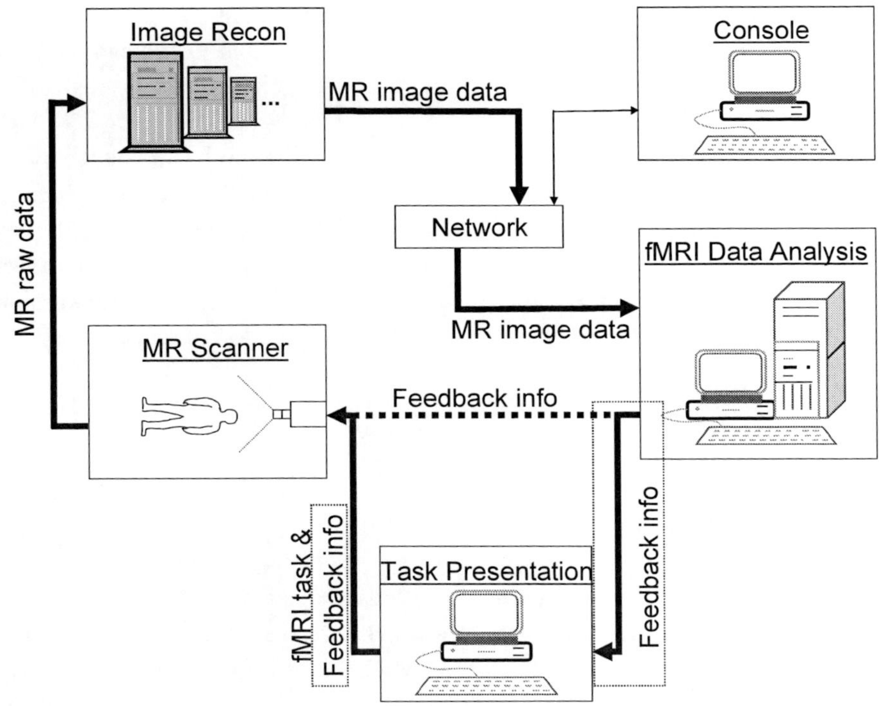

Figure 1. Schematic of a general real-time fMRI system, which is configured through close integration of the scanner, the online image reconstruction system, the task presentation system, the response monitoring system, and the online fMRI data analysis and/or real-time feedback system. The thick lines and arrows represent the data flow in real-time.

Modern scanners reconstruct the data soon after each slice is acquired. The processing may be occurring on a slice by slice basis as well, although some steps such as 3D motion correction may require a full set of slices. If the processing is complete before the next TR is complete, thus leaving enough time for next TR's data to be processed itself during the TR after that, for our purposes we shall consider it done in real-time.

Given the extra hardware, software and setup requirements of rtfMRI, one might question the advantage of rtfMRI over traditional acquisition and processing. The largest gain is in a clinical setting. It is not uncommon for fMRI researchers to discard subject's data because of data quality, often related to motion.

For a clinical scan of a patient, an immediate feedback of the quality, results and compliance of an fMRI scan is an enormous benefit. Real-time fMRI also opens intriguing biofeedback experiments for researchers, where subjects would receive information about the experiment, for example their brain's activation or their head position, in real-time. Finally, one can imagine creating dynamic experiment where the task itself changes as a result of a subject's neuronal activity.

In the remainder of this chapter, we will describe the basic concepts and technical solution of rtfMRI, with a focus on a technique that we have recently developed and implemented on a Siemens 3T MRI scanner. We will then elaborate on the potential applications of rtfMRI techniques mentioned above. In particular, we present a novel method of voluntary head-motion suppression using the feedback of the subject's own motion information in real time.

IMPLEMENTATION

Hardware Requirements and Data Flow

For conventional fMRI, the scanner and associated raw (or image) data storage facilities and task presentation system are the necessary parts of the hardware configuration. To perform fMRI in real-time, generally more stringent requirements must be met. The real-time fMRI hardware system is generally configured through close integration of the scanner, the online image reconstruction system, the task presentation system, the response monitoring system, and the online fMRI data analysis and/or real-time feedback system [8,9]. Additional hardware may be required for some specific real-time fMRI applications. Figure 1 shows a generic schematic of a real-time fMRI system with the parts in the boxes with dashed lines only for the implementation of feedback.

The real-time fMRI hardware determines the associated data flow during the fMRI experiments. The raw MR k-space (frequency space) data are acquired using the MR scanner and the raw data will immediately be transferred, via a fast connection such as an optical link, to a computer that is typically used exclusively for the image reconstruction due to the intensive computational load, especially for image reconstruction of whole-brain fMRI time series. Upon reconstruction, the image data are transferred slice by slice, or volume by volume, via internal network or local area network (LAN), to another computer which is running the real-time software. This software may be the public-domain AFNI [10], commercial software such as Turbo-Brain Voyager [11], or, most-commonly, custom-made software [8,12]. The real-time software is used for analyzing the fMRI image data, including various preprocessing steps, i.e., head motion detection and correction, detrending, and statistical analysis to get the activation maps. The intermediate analysis results, such as head motion parameters [12], activation maps [9,13] or activation intensity curves [13,14] can be simultaneously transferred to an independent feedback system for real-time presentation to the subject, or integrated into the task presentation system [12], making the fMRI experiments interactive by manipulating the ongoing paradigms according to the subject's responses. Additionally, the investigator and/or scanner operator can monitor the motion and activation of the subject [15], and stop the scan if the motion is excessive or if the activation has reached sufficient statistical power.

Image Reconstruction

In real-time fMRI experiments online image reconstruction follows immediately after the raw k-space data are sent out from the scanner. As one of the most computationally intensive tasks in real-time data processing, online image reconstruction requires powerful computer resources, often multiprocessor computers or even a cluster of PCs [15], to obtain sufficient processing speed. This is especially true for whole-brain studies. Besides hardware, image reconstruction algorithms strongly depend on the chosen fast imaging technique for fMRI data acquisition, such as single-shot echo-planar imaging (EPI) [8,12,13,14,16] or spiral imaging [17,18]. Spiral imaging acquires data along a spiral trajectory in k-space. The typical spiral image reconstruction algorithm first interpolates the raw spiral data onto an orthogonal, equidistant grid (so-called 'regridding') before a two-dimensional fast Fourier transformation [19]. In contrast, EPI acquires the raw data on a rectangular grid in k-space, therefore no regridding is necessary for EPI image reconstruction. Strategies to reduce the image reconstruction time commonly use parallel processing. Goddard et al. reported an fMRI system which includes the online image reconstruction using multiple parallel platforms [20]. Frank et al. distributed different volumes of data on different processors for image reconstruction and registration in parallel [18]. These arrangements substantially reduce the total image reconstruction time. For real-time fMRI studies, finishing all of the associated processing steps on one volume of data within the time window of one TR is necessary to achieve real-time imaging, which indirectly determines the upper limit of the time available for image reconstruction.

Motion Analysis and Correction

In fMRI data analysis, the signal intensity time series in each voxel are evaluated using various statistical methods. This is generally done under either the assumption that the subject's head remained motionless or that any residual motion can be accounted for in the statistical analysis with covariates. However, for most experiments, this is not the case [21, 22]. Subjects move substantially due to long scan times, unease over experimental procedures, orienting to experimental stimuli, swallowing, blood drawing or drug administration, or other experimental measures performed during data acquisition [12]. Although the absolute magnitudes of head movement in fMRI data are small, commonly within 1 mm, the influence of head motion cannot be ignored. The BOLD signal change generally is very small, i.e., usually 1-3% at 1.5 T magnetic field strength. If two adjacent voxels have 20% difference in their intensities (for example a gray matter voxel adjacent to a white matter voxel), a movement of 0.375 mm (10% of the voxel size of 3.75 mm, a typical image resolution in fMRI studies) will bring about 2% signal change, the same level as the BOLD signal change due to the neuronal activation [23]. If uncorrected, this motion-induced change to the voxel time series will lead to erroneous statistical inference. Depending upon the type of motion, false-positives/increased activation (for task-correlated motion) or false-negatives/decreased statistical significance (task-independent motion) volume will result, respectively. In other words, head motion will reduce the sensitivity and specificity of fMRI data analysis.

To combat this motion, image registration is normally used for motion detection and correction in fMRI data analysis [24,25]. Nearly all fMRI image registration techniques use the rigid body model, which assumes that the brain is rigid and does not deform due to head motion, breathing, and heart beat [26]. This is a reasonable assumption, although there does exist some brain motion and deformation, but only with a small amplitude in the cortex [24]. Non-rigid body models exist, but are far too computationally demanding for real-time applications.

The rigid body transformation in three-dimension (3D) space is described with six parameters, three translational parameters and three rotational parameters [24,25]. For image registration, a cost function is first defined as the measure of dissimilarity between the images, and then the transformation parameters are determined by minimizing the cost function. A least-squares criterion is widely used, where the cost function is defined as the square of the global difference between the reference image $I(\boldsymbol{r})$ and the source image $J(\boldsymbol{r})$ [24,27],

$$\sum_{r}\left|(\mathrm{T}(r)) - J(r)^2\right|, \tag{1}$$

where $\mathbf{T}$ stands for the rigid body transformation, which, in theory, can be calculated using any technique for a multi-dimensional nonlinear least-squares problem [28]. However, these commonly used techniques are extremely time-consuming and thus inappropriate for real-time application. So special treatments targeted at reducing the computation time while maintaining sufficient motion estimation accuracy are needed for the associated implementation in real-time fMRI. If the motion is small and the volumes are spatially smooth (by blurring if necessary), Eq. (1) can be linearized through expanding the source image as a first order Taylor series about the reference with respect to six rigid body transformation parameters [24,26,29]

$$J(\boldsymbol{r}) \approx I(\boldsymbol{r}) + \nabla I(\boldsymbol{r}) \cdot \boldsymbol{m} = I(\boldsymbol{r}) + \begin{pmatrix} \frac{\partial I(\boldsymbol{r}_1)}{\partial m_1} & \cdots & \frac{\partial I(\boldsymbol{r}_1)}{\partial m_6} \\ \vdots & \ddots & \vdots \\ \frac{\partial I(\boldsymbol{r}_n)}{\partial m_1} & \cdots & \frac{\partial I(\boldsymbol{r}_n)}{\partial m_6} \end{pmatrix} \cdot \begin{pmatrix} m_1 \\ \vdots \\ m_6 \end{pmatrix} \tag{2}$$

where $m_1, \cdots, m_6$ are the rigid body transformation parameters. The linear equation, Eq. (2), can be solved iteratively with repeated "reslicing" of the volume in each intermediate step, providing the estimation of six rigid body transformation parameters when the iteration converges [24].

As stated before, for real-time applications the convergence of the iteration has to be rapid. Solving the linear equation, Eq. (2), is straightforward, so the key is how to more efficiently "reslice" or regrid the volume into new intermediate grid positions in each iterative step, which, to a great extent, determines the total calculation time and precision [30,31]. If only the computational speed is considered, simple linear interpolation of the volume to the new grid is the best. However, image blurring will result, which will degrade image quality and potentially impair the convergence. In contrary, sinc interpolation is the best for image quality [24,27], but is costly in terms of calculation time. Recently, a few new processing strategies have been proposed for this problem [23, 26, 30, 32].

As proposed by Eddy et al. [30], if regridding is performed in k-space, much lower computation load can be achieved while maintaining sufficient accuracy. This is due to the following reasons. First, a shift in image space (or i-space) is equivalent to simple phase multiplications in k-space according to the Fourier shift theorem. Second, rotation in i-space also corresponds to rotation in k-space; however, a rotation can be approximated by successive shearing operations. Shearing operations are realized through column/row-wise translations, which still can exploit the Fourier shift theorem in k-space to replace the translations with phase multiplications. As a result, "quite accurate approximation with only a moderate amount of computation" of rotation and shifting (translation) operations is achieved [30]. Cox et al. expanded Eddy's 2D shearing operation directly to 3D, which further speeded up the computation [23, 26]. The interested audience can refer to the references [23, 26, 30, 32] for the details. Using the above methods, an accurate real-time motion detection and correction can be achieved in an expedient fashion, leaving some time for real-time analysis of the fMRI data.

Statistical Analysis

The overriding issues in real-time fMRI statistical analysis parallel those of registration in many ways. Besides registration there are a number of steps in typical offline fMRI analysis such as distortion correction, spatial filtering, spatial normalization to a standard space and temporal filtering. These steps are a prelude to the statistical modeling, which is usually some variation of the general linear model (GLM) [29]. However, other more sophisticated, and computationally demanding, multivariate techniques are becoming more popular such as independent component analysis (ICA) [33] or partial least squares [34]. Unfortunately, many of these preprocessing steps and analysis methods are too time consuming to be practical for real-time fMRI. It is likely that this will always be the case – as computational resources increase, so will the complexity of the most sophisticated analysis as researchers are generally willing to expend that time. For real-time applications some steps must be omitted and some simplifications to the analysis or algorithm improvements must be made.

Some groups make a distinction between real-time and 'online' (sometime called 'in-time' or 'near real-time') analysis, the latter being finishing the analysis soon after the completion of the scan. Goddard et al. [20] used a variety of parallel computing platforms to complete a complicate processing stream including spiral reconstruction, motion correction, regridding and statistical analysis. This was done using the 'FIASCO' software package.

Offline analysis steps are typically designed to operate on an entire dataset at once (e.g., all of the slices in one image or all of the time points in a voxel). Thus as the number of time points increase so does the calculation time, eventually reaching a point where real-time processing becomes impossible. One solution is to operate only on the last N time points – the so-called 'sliding window' analysis used in software such as 'FIRE' [35,36]. This has the added advantage of being dynamic in the sense that the activation maps can change over the course of an experiment – a necessary condition for some real-time applications like neurofeedback, discussed below. Additionally, sliding-window analysis would be necessary for examining the dynamics of activation associated with changes in cognitive strategy and tasks that would take advantage of these changes and modify the stimuli based upon the activation. In contrast, one can imagine applications where real-time functional maps based upon the entire time course, the so-call cumulative approach, such as clinical scans where scanning to a criterion, such as a given region of the brain activating, is appropriate. With this approach the number of false-positives decreases with time, at the expense of losing the ability to see changes in activation with time.

Cox et al. [37] were the first group to perform real-time analysis using the entire time course, which is integrated into the AFNI analysis suite [10]. They modified the calculation of correlation coefficients to be calculated incrementally – that is each new image modifies the previously calculated correlation coefficient. They also include optional removal of nuisance terms such as a mean and linear trend. Cohen similarly reports an incremental correlation approach [8]. Others, such as Voyvodic et al. [38] calculate t-statistics in an incremental fashion. Their software package, FSCAN, then calculates a more complicated model including cardiac and respiratory effects at the end of scanning. The advantage of using correlation over a t-statistic is that the former allows for a reference vector whose shape varies with time. This is critical for so-called event-related experiments where the stimuli are brief compared to the hemodynamic response such that each event is expected to result in a hemodynamic response. The above approaches are limited in that they produce a single statistical quantity. Whereas that may be sufficient for simple designs that may occur in clinical settings, in current fMRI research there are typically several conditions in each run, with the data processed using GLM. By using a least-squares algorithm designed for limited computation time and memory, Smyster et al. were able to achieve real-time analysis and display for high-resolution EPI (128x128), but a limited number of slices/brain volume [39]. The speed depended on both the number of voxels and the number of regressors. A notable feature of their approach is the incorporation of an input mask and an output mask. The former restricts data aggregation to intracerebral voxels – reducing memory and computational costs, and the later restricts where the regression parameters and statistics are computed, again reducing computational costs. The output mask can be changed during the experiment without any computational penalty. Using a cluster of PCs, Bagarinao et al. were able to perform a comprehensive processing pipeline including realignment, smoothing and a full GLM model in real-time [15]. Their cluster consisted of 16 nodes using off-the-shelf PC components. The GLM coefficients were computed using a recursive algorithm that permitted incremental calculations that they implemented [40]. Using this system, they were able to process a 30 slice 64x64 dataset in just over 1 second and a 20 slice 128x128 dataset in just over 2.5 seconds. As mentioned earlier, one of the most promising multivariate analysis approaches is independent components analysis (ICA). ICA is a non-hypothesis driven approach which decomposes fMRI data into independent spatial maps, each associated with a component timecourse. Until recently, it has been used exclusively for offline analysis. However, Esposito et al. demonstrated a real-time analysis strategy using ICA [41]. They used a limited subset of time points in a sliding-window fashion, but cleverly averaged the sliding-window maps of the component of interest to create an accurate cumulative map. One of its complications is choosing the component(s) of interest. This group used a ROI approach where the experimenter chooses a brain region expected to be activated, and the program automatically chooses the component most active in that region. Unfortunately, their implementation precluded full-brain imaging as even a single slice (128x128) could take greater than one second to process.

APPLICATIONS

Due to its incomparable power in detecting brain functions noninvasively with high sensitivity and spatial specificity, the use of fMRI has increased dramatically in recent years [8, 38]. Real-time implementation of fMRI greatly enhances the utility of this technique in various aspects. We will discuss, in this section, applications of rtfMRI in quality assurance, interactive manipulation of tasks, biofeedback, and a detailed example of head-motion reduction using online feedback of subject's own head motion information.

Quality Assurance and Interactive Control

At the simplest level, routine real-time fMRI can be used to assure data quality by having the scan operator stop the scan if the online analysis indicates that the subject is performing poorly (i.e., excessive head motion, or misunderstanding the instructions, etc.) and reacquire the data before the subject leaves the scanner. The MRI environment – the confined space, constricting restraints and loud noises – can easily distract the subjects from the task at hand. Additionally, subjects simply don't have sufficient proprioception to detect the minute motions that critically affect the fMRI data, especially when the subject is occupied with the task. Information from rtfMRI can be used to evaluate whether the paradigm is followed by the subject or if the research aim has been reached, during the scan or at least while the subject remains in the scanner bore [15, 18]. This ability to 'scan to criteria' could be a great benefit to clinical scans like pre-surgical mapping where one must collect sufficient data to define a certain functional region of the brain. Online analysis also makes it possible for investigator to manipulate the paradigm for subsequent scans according to the analysis results of the ongoing scan. With interactive real-time paradigm control and online fMRI analysis, fMRI experiments will become more flexible and the data reliability will be improved. The subjects will benefit from this technique as well, especially for patients with neurological and/or psychiatric disorder where monitoring is strongly needed in the scanner [18, 38].

Biofeedback and Self-Regulation

Biofeedback is a technique of monitoring one's own physiological parameters, such as heart rate, skin temperature, skin conductance, and specific frequency components of brainwaves, therefore gaining a certain level of voluntary manipulation or self-regulation of these biological measures by conscious mental control [9, 13]. Among the various applications of biofeedback, there is a more specific area that targets the self-regulation of a subject's own brain function with EEG (electroencephalogram) biofeedback, also know as "neurofeedback" [9]. Training and therapeutic intervention with EEG neurofeedback are commonly applied in clinical practice for improving brain functions such as "concentration, short term memory, speech, motor skills, sleep, energy level, and emotional balance." [42] The high temporal resolution (on the order of a millisecond) achieved by EEG neurofeedback makes it easy to measure rapid changes in electrical brain activity and give immediate feedback. However, the source localization capability of EEG is limited. Since EEG electrodes are put on the scalp, in theory EEG signals collected come from a large volume of the brain. Due to the spatial smearing and various potential interferences in the large brain volume, EEG neurofeedback is mainly limited to autonomic and global physiological parameters, and thus traditionally is used for improving relaxation, attention and other generic behaviors that involve global brain process not tied to specific brain regions [17,42].

While EEG neurofeedback is still widely implemented, a new, more powerful, spatially constrained neurofeedback technique, fMRI-based neurofeedback, has been developed recently, which exploits the greater spatial localization capability inherent in magnetic resonance imaging [9,42]. Because the information derived from fMRI is required to be fed back during ongoing scan, shortly after each trial, or at least before subjects leave the MR scanner, the advent of this new type of neurofeedback greatly depends on the fMRI data acquisition and processing techniques. These have improved considerably in recent years, including increased gradient power and higher magnetic field strength allowing for faster MR imaging with an adequate signal-to-noise ratio (SNR), and faster computers and data processing software providing the possibility of reconstructing images and performing statistical analysis in real-time [13]. In other words, real-time fMRI lays down the technical basis for fMRI-based neurofeedback.

One of the first feasibility studies for fMRI-based neurofeedback was reported by Yoo and Jolesz [9], where they developed an fMRI infrastructure with a neurofeedback capability. In that study, the subjects were presented with visual feedback of their own brain activation maps during a motor task. It was demonstrated that neurofeedback successfully guided the subjects to expand the activation in the motor and somatosensory cortex. The subjects adjusted their motor strategies with the help of feedback, although the feedback was delayed approximately 20 s after the completion of each movement trial, therefore not exactly in real time [9]. Another fMRI neurofeedback study used a self-induced sadness task with randomized presentation of sad or neutral faces in each trial, 10 trials per scan [36]. The level of the neuronal activation in the amygdala, a main brain region involved in the response to the negative mood, was fed back to the subjects in each trial to enhance the induction of sadness. Although the study, as pointed out by other researchers [13,17], didn't try to separate the effects due to the feedback from the effects due to the visual presentation of sad facial expressions, it did demonstrate the capability of online feedback of fMRI information to the subjects [36]. In another study, researchers [13] directly fed back the local BOLD signals of the targeted brain region to the subjects in a time series, similar with the use of brain waves in EEG biofeedback. They emphasized the importance of immediate feedback (less than 2-second delay following the data acquisition), considering that in EEG neurofeedback minimum delays facilitate self-regulation [13]. The sole subject in that study successfully increased and decreased his own local BOLD signals following the task instructions, and the achieved BOLD-response was reported to increase with the help of feedback training. The revealed training effect suggested the potential of voluntary control of the circumscribed brain region using fMRI-based neurofeedback [13]. A more recent report represented the first full study of training a group of subjects to control their brain activation in a local brain region using real-time fMRI neurofeedback [17]. The subjects performed an imagined manual action task and were asked to achieve a dynamically-updated activation level in the target brain region with the help of real-time feedback of their current activation in that brain region. The voluntary control of the brain activation was enhanced in the group of subjects receiving the fMRI neurofeedback compared with the control group without neurofeedback. The brain activation in the subjects receiving feedback reached the same level in the imagined manual action task as when the subjects performed actual manual action. These effects of voluntary control continued even after fMRI neurofeedback was removed. This study systematically proved the possibility of the mental control of activation over the circumscribed regions using real-time fMRI neurofeedback.

Motion Reduction

Subject head motion is a common problem in fMRI experiments [21, 22]. Although various physical restraints including a bite bar, supporting pillows or compression pads are routinely used at most facilities, the problem remains with a significant cost of lost data. The common methods for dealing with moderate head motion, "retrospective" motion correction using image registration in post-processing [23,29,32,43,44,45] and "prospective" motion correction during ongoing scanning [26,46,47,48,49,50], are successful to varying degrees with some remaining motion artifacts [25,51]. Preventing motion during data acquisition is still preferred [12]. Real-time monitoring of the subject head motion parameters using online image registration has proved to be a very useful quality assurance (QA) tool [23]. If the estimated movements are too large, the subjects may be re-scanned immediately. However, the method is not suitable for many studies, such as the studies involving learning and/or practice effects, or drug administration, where a repeated acquisition would confound the experimental manipulations [12]. It is observed in practice that verbal feedback from investigators between scan runs can help to reduce the amount of head motion significantly. Most subjects simply don't have a good proprioceptive feel for how still they need to remain, or how much movement they are making in the magnet [23]. However, the feedback in this way is very operator dependent. In the last section of the chapter, we demonstrate a specific application of real-time fMRI – a voluntary head-motion suppression method by consistent feedback to subjects of their own head motion information in real time [12]. The method was tested in two sets of experiments, the original design [52], herein called as Design I, and an improved design [12], herein called as Design II. In Design I, subjects watched six head motion curves in a full screen while performing an auditory verbal N-BACK task. In Design II, the feedback of head motion information was simplified to a visual cue shown within a visual N-BACK task. A real-time fMRI analysis system was developed for the above purposes on standard MR imaging hardware. The real-time fMRI analysis system was developed on a Siemens 3T Allegra head-only scanner (Siemens, Erlangen, Germany). In Design I, the system hardware, involving the scanner HOST computer, the MRIR (MR Image Reconstruction) computer and the RT (real-time analysis) computer, are connected to each other in an internal network. The system software involves an ICE (Image Calculation Environment) program that we developed for real-time image reconstruction and image transfer and the AFNI package [10] for real-time motion correction and functional analysis.

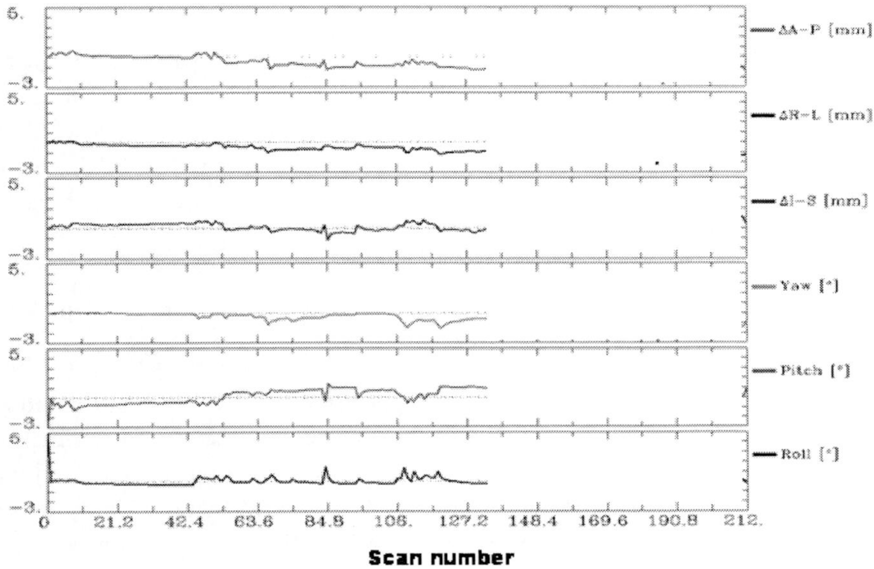

Figure 2. An example of six head motion curves shown in a whole screen, through which the subject could watch his (or her) own head motion status while he or she was performing an auditory N-BACK task. The six motion parameters, ΔA-P, ΔR-L, ΔI-S, Yaw, Pitch and Roll are the output of the AFNI real-time plug-in.

The ICE program achieves the parallel processing of image reconstruction and image transfer with data acquisition. Upon reconstruction of one slice on the MRIR computer, the image is sent using TCP/IP sockets to the RT computer where AFNI waits for incoming data with its real-time plug-in. After each 3D volume is complete, online image registration is evoked, and the estimated motion parameters are displayed in a continually updating graph on the monitor of the server. The graph is also simultaneously displayed on the screen in the scanner bore that subjects can watch during the ongoing scan, as shown in Figure 2. The data transfer and motion parameter calculation are finished within about 100ms, much less than a TR. Due to parallel processing between the data acquisition and data processing, accurate real-time 3D registration and motion display are achieved. Online activation analysis can also be performed with this system, although it was not used in this study [52].

An auditory N-BACK paradigm was used in Design I. Auditory stimuli were presented in 30-s epochs to subjects via an air-conduction tube. Condition A is a rest period. During the epochs of 1-BACK (Condition B) and 2-BACK (Condition C), subjects listen to a series of 15 neutral words with an interstimulus interval of 2 s. Cycles of alternation between conditions were pseudorandomized within the 9 minute scan, e.g., ABCACBABCACBACBA. The N-BACK tasks were repeated in three scenarios with the subjects watching the their own real head motion curves (Real-Curve), watching the fake head motion curves (Fake-Curve, data from another subject) and without watching any curves (No-Curve). A head motion index is defined from the 6 motion parameters that AFNI outputs, ΔA-P, ΔR-L, ΔI-S, Yaw, Pitch and Roll (see Figure 2), i.e., $\sqrt{d_1^2+d_2^2+d_3^2+r_1^2\theta_1^2+r_2^2\theta_2^2+r_3^2\theta_3^2}$, where d_i and θ_i stand for the three translational and the three rotational parameters, respectively, and $\boldsymbol{r_i}$ stands for the mean rotational semi-radii around the three directions. The head motion index, the performance accuracy and reaction time, and the activation map were evaluated. The experiments were performed on five healthy control subjects at our site and the subjects gave written informed consent for participation in this IRB-approved study. Thirty-seven sagittal slices were acquired using a 2D EPI-BOLD pulse sequences with TR=2500 ms, TE=27 ms, matrix size = 64×64, FOV = 220 mm, slice thickness/gap = 4/0 mm, flip angle = 80°, bandwidth = 3552 Hz/pixel, measurement # = 212.

Scan Number (TR)

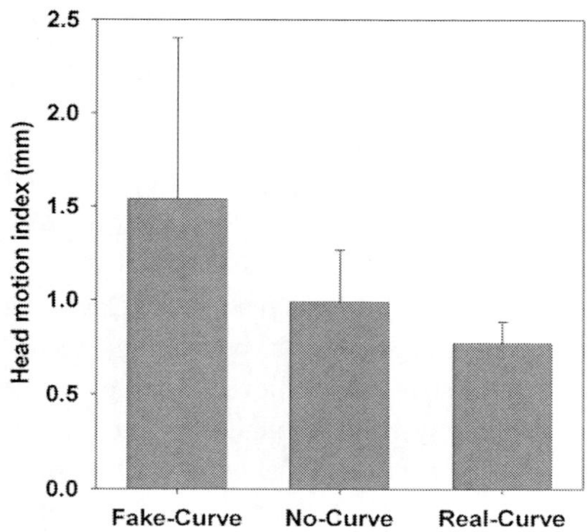

Figure 3. The mean head motion indexes for five subjects under the three scenarios, i.e., Fake-Curve, No-Curve, and Real-Curve, respectively. A reduction in head motion was seen as subjects watched their own head motion curves.

The mean head motion indexes under the three scenarios are shown in Figure 3. A reduction in head motion due to watching the real motion curves was seen, compared with the other two conditions, i.e., Fake_Curve and No_Curve. The performance accuracy was analyzed using two-way repeated-measures ANOVA where $F(2, 6) = 2.256$, $p = 0.186$ for the main effect of feedback. The same procedure was repeated for the reaction time where $F(2, 6) = 7.568$, $p = 0.023$. No significant differences were found in performance accuracy but there was a significant increase in reaction time. The group analyses of the functional MRI data were carried out offline using the 3dANOVA2 program of AFNI. Figure 4 is the map of activation difference between No-Curve and Real-Curve with $p<0.001$ (*unadjusted*). Differences in brain activation are seen in the lateral frontal and posterior parietal regions that are closely related to the working memory task. The feedback of motion curves in this study significantly influences brain activation and reaction time of the N-BACK task, even though no effects on performance accuracy are observed. Thus it appears that the voluntary motion control may serve as a secondary cognitive task and alter the response to the primary cognitive task. Therefore, improvements of the motion suppression method are necessary to minimize the interference on the primary fMRI task. These results led to an improved design, i.e., Design II. In Design II, the feedback of head motion information was simplified to a visual cue shown within a visual N-BACK task [12]. An additional computer, for integrating the head motion feedback information into the fMRI task and presenting both to subjects, i.e., the TASK computer, is added to the hardware components of the real-time fMRI system in Design II. The HOST, the MRIR and the RT computer were interconnected on an internal network via 100 Mbps Ethernet. The RT computer is connected to the TASK computer via RS-232 serial ports. The hardware components form a closed loop in which the MR raw data originate from the subject and the final head motion information estimated from the image data is fed back to the subject. The added software components of the real-time fMRI system in Design II include a separate program we developed on the RT computer for communications between a modified real-time plug-in in AFNI and the TASK computer, and a modified visual N-BACK task on the TASK computer written in E-Prime (Psychology Software Tools Inc., Pittsburgh, PA). The motion parameters are displayed on the RT computer monitor in a continually updating graph similar to the one the subject saw in Design I – see Figure 2. This graph permits the investigator to observe subject head motion. Additionally, AFNI sends the data via UNIX sockets to the separate program mentioned above on the RT computer, which simply collects that motion data and sends it out through a serial port to the TASK computer, where the head motion information and fMRI task are integrated and presented, as described below.

Twelve healthy right-handed male volunteers (mean age 26.9 years) participated in this experiment after giving written informed consent to this IRB-approved study. The modified version of the visual N-BACK task consists of six 4'12" runs in a pseudo-randomized block design. Each run consists of one block each of 1, 2 and 3-BACK conditions (15 stimuli per block), separated by blocks of 0-BACK (control condition, 9 stimuli per block). The stimuli are letters, each presented for 500 ms with an inter-stimulus interval (ISI) of 2500 ms.

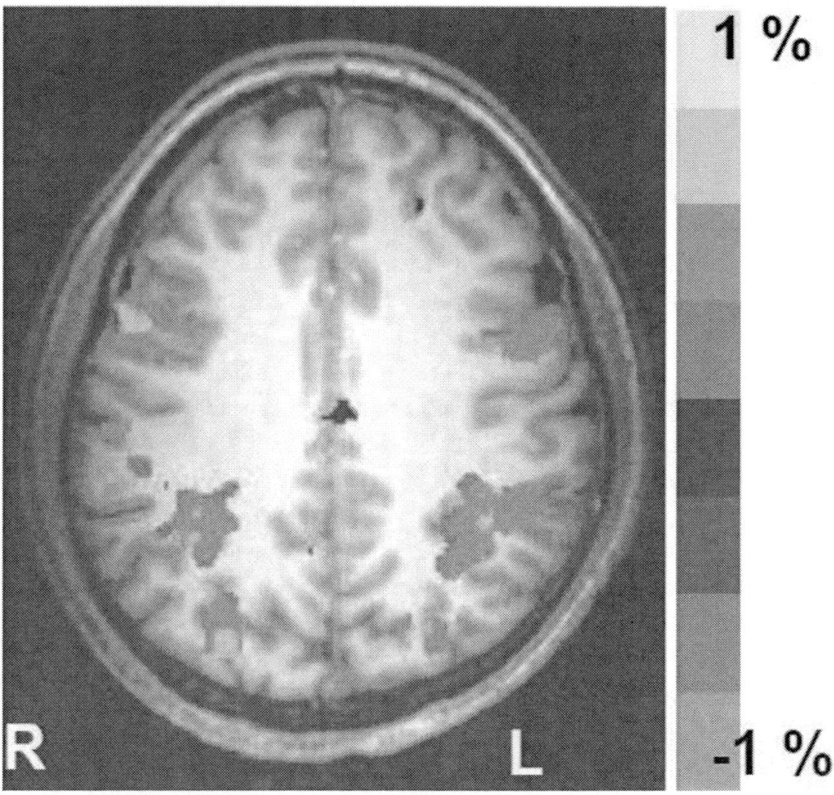

Figure 4. Map of activation difference between No-Curve and Real-Curve with $p < 0.001$ (*unadjusted*). Differences in brain activation are seen in the regions that are closely related to the working memory task, such as the lateral frontal and posterior parietal regions. The color bar in the right shows the BOLD signal difference as a percentage change from baseline.

Our typical visual N-BACK task was modified to include the following new functions: reading the serial port for online head motion information, updating of motion feedback information, and synchronizing with the scanner. Motion information was conveyed to the subject via a group of arrows on the display (see Figure 5). During much of the ISI and instruction screens, the task polled the serial port for current motion information and updated the arrow group accordingly. To maintain accurate timing, resynchronization with the scanner was repeated each TR.

Each subject repeated the modified N-BACK tasks under two conditions in a counterbalanced design, once with feedback of the head motion information (MotFB) and once without feedback of the head motion information (No_MotFB). The two scenarios occurred in one session, one immediately after the other. The head motion information was displayed as a four-way arrow group changing color from green to red when a composite head motion index went beyond a specified threshold, which is detailed below. In the No_MotFB condition, the color of the arrow group remained the same (blue) at all times, irrespective of the subjects' motion. For the MotFB experiment, subjects were informed to observe any changes in the arrows, to try to stay still, especially if the arrows changed, but to not compensate for any motion. Critically, before each task, subjects were informed that the most important thing was to stay focused on the task and secondarily to be aware of arrow changes with their peripheral vision. They were further informed that the colors would change back to green just by them keeping still. No directional significance for the arrows was implied in the instructions and given that all four directions changed simultaneously (see Figure 5), it was impossible for subjects to infer a direction and try and compensate for the motion. For both conditions, subjects were told to stay as still as possible at all times. On a Siemens 3T Allegra head-only scanner, whole-brain scanning was performed using a 2D EPI pulse sequence with 39 sagittal slices, TR = 3000 ms, TE = 27 ms, matrix size = 64×64, FOV = 220 mm, slice thickness/gap = 4/0 mm, flip angle = 85º, bandwidth = 4112 Hz per pixel, number of measurements per run = 84. Additionally, 1 mm^3 resolution T1 weighted structural scans were obtained for spatial normalization using a MPRAGE pulse sequence. The head motion feedback information was integrated into the fMRI task by presenting the arrow group along with the visual N-BACK task. The arrow group, along with the visual N-BACK stimuli, was back-projected onto a screen above the subject's head by a LCD projector, which the subjects viewed via a mirror. The letters and the fixation were displayed at the center of the screen.

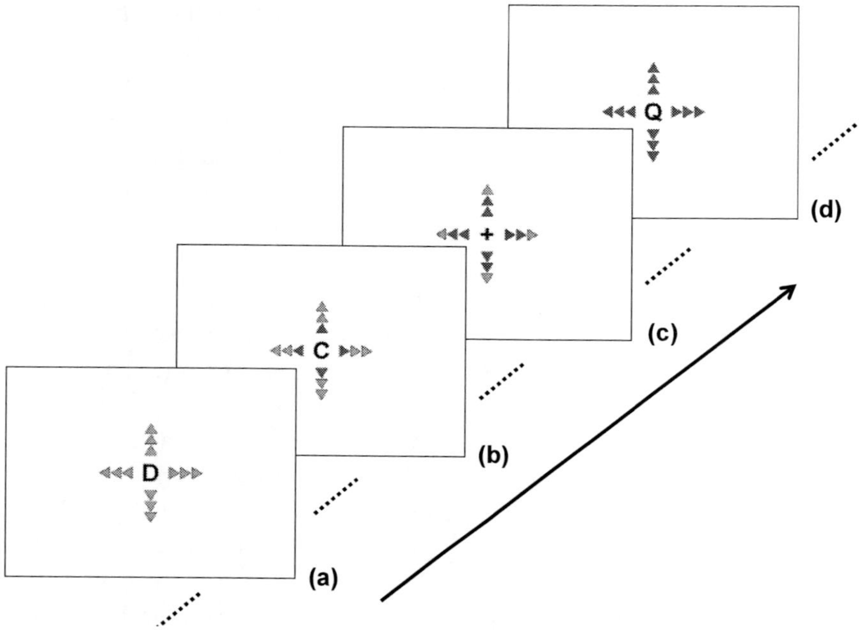

Figure 5. Example screens from the N-BACK task along with the four-way arrow group at different states based upon the value of the motion index, $M(t)$ in Eq. (3): (a) $M(t) < 0.2$ mm (b) 0.2 mm $< M(t) <$ 0.4 mm, (c) 0.4 mm $< M(t) <$ 0.6 mm, (d) $M(t) >$ 0.6 mm.

The four-way arrow group surrounded the screen center in the four perpendicular directions in the arrangement shown in Figure 5. The arrow group sections, the inner (I), middle (II) and outer (III), were related to three empirically derived thresholds based on the head motion index described below. When a subject's head motion index was below the 1st threshold, all three sections were green Figure 5a. When the head motion index went beyond the 1st threshold but below the 2nd threshold, Section I turned red Figure 5b. Sections II and III turned red analogously when the 2nd and 3rd threshold were exceeded, respectively Figure 5c-d.

The head motion index is defined as

$$M(t) = w\,M(t - \Delta t) + \Delta MOT \qquad (3)$$

where ΔMOT is written as

$$\Delta MOT = \sqrt{\begin{matrix}[m_1(t) - m_1(t-\Delta t)]^2 + [m_2(t) - m_2(t-\Delta t)]^2 + [m_3(t) - m_3(t-\Delta t)]^2 \\ + r_\theta^2[m_4(t) - m_4(t-\Delta t)]^2 + r_\phi^2[m_5(t) - m_5(t-\Delta t)]^2 + r_\varphi^2[m_6(t) - m_6(t-\Delta t)]^2\end{matrix}}$$

and $\Delta t = 1$ TR. This is the total amount of head motion between two adjacent TRs, where $m_1(t)$, $m_2(t)$, and $m_3(t)$ are the three translational parameters, $m_4(t)$, $m_5(t)$, and $m_6(t)$ are the three rotational parameters, and r_θ, r_ϕ, and r_φ are the semi-radii around the three axes. Eq. (3) is a typical recurrent expression, which gives a weight, w, of 1 to the motion that just happened, ΔMOT, and a weight of less than 1 to the previous motion, $M(t-\Delta t)$. Based upon analysis of historic data, the three empirical thresholds were set as 0.2, 0.4, and 0.6 mm, respectively.

FMRI image analysis was performed using AFNI. Data were preprocessed with retrospective motion correction. Motion curves from this step were analyzed two ways to determine the effectiveness of head motion suppression. Figure 6 shows the mean number per session of greater than 0.2 mm head motion indices under the two scenarios. Mean head motion counts decreased significantly from a mean of 39.41 (No_MotFB) to a mean of 11.08 (MotFB) (Z=3.059, p=0.002), shown as the thick line and two big black dots. This head motion suppression was seen in every subject, shown as the thin lines and small black dots. A histogram of composite online head motion index, calculated from Eq. (3), along time in one run was evaluated for the MotFB and No_MotFB conditions. The histogram (shown in Figure 7) represents the number of motion excursions above 0.2 mm as a function of time, which is obtained by summing the number at each time point across 6 runs for each subject, then averaged across subjects. Examination of the histogram shows that task-related head motion was suppressed in the MotFB condition. Head motion data and behavioral data were analyzed with repeated-measures ANOVA and nonparametric Wilcoxon signed ranks tests using SPSS (SPSS Inc., Chicago, IL, USA).

No significant differences were found in the behavioral data between the MotFB and No_MotFB conditions. For accuracy, results of a 2 (feedback) X 4 (N-BACK task level) MANOVA were $F_{1,11} = 3.157$, $p = 0.10$ (n.s.) for a main effect of feedback and $F_{3,33} = 1.916$, $p = 0.146$ (n.s.) for the feedback X task interaction. Similar analysis for reaction time yielded $F_{1,11} = 2.497$, $p = 0.142$ (n.s.) for a main effect of feedback and $F_{3,33} = 2.046$, $p = 0.126$ (n.s.) for the feedback X task interaction. Results of voxel-wise analysis of brain activation indicated no significant difference between the MotFB and No_MotFB conditions. A more sensitive region of interest (ROI) analysis over 38 brain regions activated by the task found no regions with a significant feedback X task interaction and only 2 regions that had a significant main effect of feedback at $p < 0.05$, *uncorrected.* Interestingly, the two significant regions, posterior cingulate ($F_{1,11} = 5.281$, $p = 0.042$) and right superior temporal gyrus ($F_{1,11} = 5.5$, $p = 0.039$) were both regions that were *deactivated* by the N-BACK task. In both regions, there was less deactivation in the MotFB condition. There is evidence that deactivation is more related to internal processing during rest than being task driven. The ROI map and average activation for 2 regions, including the posterior cingulate, are shown in Figure 8. In this section we demonstrated a new strategy, to address head motion confounds, that depends critically on the ability of rtfMRI to preprocess the data in real-time such that parameters of the processing can be feed back to the subject. Significant reduction in mean head motion was observed, along with a reduction of task-correlated motion. The influence on task performance and brain activation was minimal. The current design indicates that a concise, clear, simple, non-overwhelming feedback of head motion information is the key to implementing this idea.

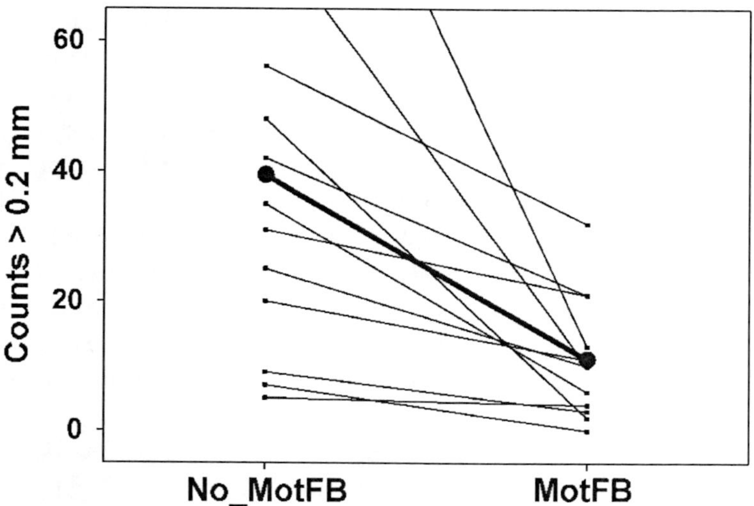

Figure 6. Mean times that the head motion index was larger than 0.2 mm with (MotFB) and without (No_MotFB) head motion feedback. The thick line and two big black dots represent the mean values for the twelve subjects, while the thin lines and small black dots are the data for each subject. Two large motion counts larger than 60 are cut off in the figure. Note that all subjects showed improvement.

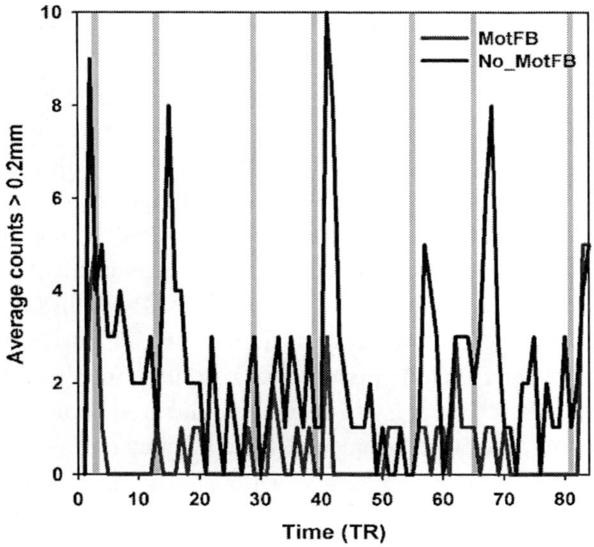

Figure 7. Histogram of counts of head motion index > 0.2 mm (from Eq. (3) with $w = 0$) along time in one run for MotFB (blue) and No_MotFB (black) conditions. Data were summed over 6 runs within subjects and then averaged across subjects. Shaded bars indicate times when instructions appeared and/or when task blocks ended. Examination of the histogram shows that task-related head motion was greatly suppressed in the MotFB condition.

It is proposed that under certain experimental conditions and subject populations, voluntary head motion suppression may feasibly be employed without significant compromise of fMRI data. The real-time fMRI system has been developed on standard MR imaging hardware. Most of the hardware components of the real-time system are part of Siemens' standard equipment; the only additional hardware is a PC running LINUX. Other than the custom set of IDEA and ICE programs, the software components are also standard. Thus, it should be fairly straightforward to implement this procedure on other platforms.

Discussion and Conclusion

FMRI has been used extensively to study the functions of the human brain. A typical fMRI experiment usually acquires several hundred brain images. The intensive computational cost inherent in fMRI data analysis makes it more reasonable to perform the analysis offline. However, immediate analysis of fMRI data has unique advantages both for neuroscience studies and clinical applications, which are the underlying fuel for the development of real-time analysis of fMRI data. As discussed in the previous sections, the advantages provided by rtfMRI include more effective QA monitoring on the task performance of the subject, more flexibility in allowing interactive paradigm manipulation, immediately locating brain regions with expected activation for subsequent scans, immediate feedback of the subject's brain activity to assist the subject in achieving a certain level of mental control of his own neuronal response, for either the recovery of lost brain function or basic research on internal cognitive mechanisms. Other applications that are not detailed in this chapter include pre-surgical planning, in which rtfMRI can be used immediately before surgery to define the functional brain regions that are targeted for surgery or, more commonly, to be avoided during the operation.

With the progress of computer hardware, MR scanner facilities and fMRI data processing algorithms, more subtle applications with rtfMRI are possible, such as the case given in the last section - voluntary head motion suppression with the help of immediate feedback of subject's own head motion information. The technique itself is complicated because the feedback information is not a part of the stimuli of the normal tasks that the subjects are performing during the scan. The interference from feedback to the normal task definitely exists; however, the degree of influence may vary depending on the feedback design. While Design II in the last section minimally influenced the task performance, further investigation on any subtle influence may be beneficial before this technique is applied more widely. In contrast to conventional biofeedback of behavioral or physiological information, such as the subject's task performance accuracy, breathing or heart rate, etc., immediate feedback of the subject's own localized brain activation is only feasible with rtfMRI and several new fMRI research projects are thus possible. Mental control over localized brain activation with the help of feedback has been illustrated in a few rtfMRI reports in literature [17, 53, 54]. Until recently, the intention has been focused on feasibility studies, i.e., whether the localized brain activation can be manipulated with the feedback of brain activity (using the raw BOLD signals or activation levels) on one pre-specified brain region. The actual extent that mental control can achieve on different brain regions, such as the brain activation amplitude and spatial specificity, are unknown yet. Interesting questions like whether two regions can be simultaneously controlled with the help of feedback, or whether the subject can increase brain activation on one region and decrease those on the other region independently have yet to be addressed.

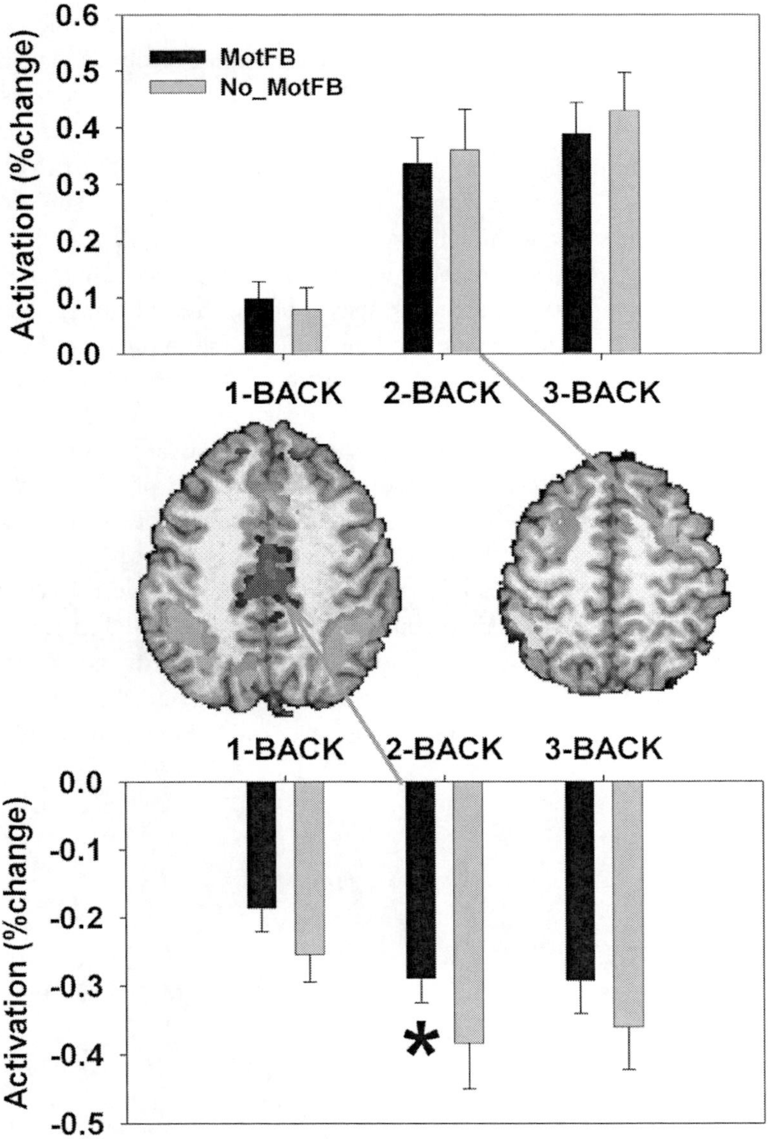

Figure 8. Regions used in a region of interest (ROI) analysis. The colors indicate the average magnitude of activation in the 3-BACK – 0-BACK contrast. The two graphs depict activation (% BOLD signal change) averaged over a given region for three task difficulties (all minus 0-BACK) with and without motion feedback (MotFB and No_MotFB, respectively). Of the regions shown, only the posterior cingulate had a significant main effect of feedback (deactivation decrease). One other region (right superior temporal gyrus) was significant for feedback; there were no significant interactions of feedback X task.

How do the other brain regions behave when the brain activation on one target region is voluntarily manipulated with the help of feedback? The answer to the above questions will help reveal the internal working mechanisms of some brain functions and even the connectivity between different brain regions. The common procedure in neurofeedback studies using rtfMRI is to instruct the subject to achieve certain levels of brain activity; the subject needs to figure out what strategies to employ to achieve this goal. A statistical study on the various strategies that the subjects have employed after successful accomplishment of the experiments may help to reveal the relationship between the various brain activities and the different brain regions. Ultimately, this kind of study will be beneficial to the patients who are receiving recovery treatment with the help of rtfMRI neurofeedback. They can adopt the same strategies that have been reported successful in activating specific brain activation to gradually restore their lost brain function, or self-regulate the disturbed brain activation. There is already preliminary evidence that this approach may be helpful for the treatment of chronic pain [54].

With continuous progress of rtfMRI, we believe that the role of rtfMRI will gradually turn from a mainly complementary tool to fMRI at present into a more complete and comparably independent sub-area in the fMRI field, which may help us to understand how the brain works more clearly in basic research and at the same time improve the associated clinical applications and benefit patients.

REFERENCES

[1] Ogawa, S., Lee, T. M., Kay, A. R. and Tank, D. W. (1990) Brain magnetic resonance imaging with contrast dependent on blood oxygenation. *Proc. Natl. Acad. Sci. USA, 87*, 9868-9872.

[2] Ogawa, S. and Lee, T. M. (1990) Magnetic resonance imaging of blood vessels at high fields: in vivo and in vitro measurements and image simulation. *Magn. Reson.Med., 16*, 9-18.

[3] Fox, P. T. and Raichle, M. E. (1986) Focal physiological uncoupling of cerebral blood flow and oxidative metabolism during somatosensory stimulation in human subjects. *Proc. Natl. Acad. Sci. USA, 83*, 1140-1144.

[4] Mansfield, P. (1977) Multi-Planar Image-Formation Using NMR Spin Echoes. *Journal of Physics C-Solid State Physics, 10*, L55-L58.

[5] Ahn, C. B., Kim, J. H. and Cho, Z. H. (1986) High-Speed Spiral-Scan Echo Planar Nmr Imaging .1. *IEEE Transactions on Medical Imaging, 5*, 2-7.

[6] Lundstrom, M. (2003) Moore's law forever? *Science, 299*, 210-211.

[7] Becker, D., Ligon, W., Merkey, P. and Ross, R. (1999) Beowulf: Low-cost supercomputing using Linux. *IEEE Software, 16*, 79-79.

[8] Cohen, M. S. (2001) Real-time functional magnetic resonance imaging. *Methods, 25*, 201-220.

[9] Yoo, S. S. and Jolesz, F. A. (2002) Functional MRI for neurofeedback: feasibility study on a hand motor task. *Neuroreport, 13*, 1377-1381.

[10] Cox, R. W. (1996) AFNI: software for analysis and visualization of functional magnetic resonance neuroimages. *Comput. Biomed. Res., 29*, 162-173.

[11] Goebel, R. (2001) Cortex-based real-time fMRI. *NeuroImage, 13*, 129-129.

[12] Yang, S., Ross, T. J., Zhang, Y., Stein, E. A. and Yang, Y. (2005) Head-Motion Suppression Using Real-Time Feedback of Motion Information and its Effects on Task Performance in fMRI. *NeuroImage, 27*, 153-162.

[13] Weiskopf, N., Veit, R., Erb, M., Mathiak, K., Grodd, W., Goebel, R. and Birbaumer, N. (2003) Physiological self-regulation of regional brain activity using real-time functional magnetic resonance imaging (fMRI): methodology and exemplary data. *NeuroImage, 19*, 577-586.

[14] Weiskopf, N., Mathiak, K., Bock, S. W., Scharnowski, F., Veit, R., Grodd, W., Goebel, R. and Birbaumer, N. (2004) Principles of a brain-computer interface (BCI) based on real-time functional magnetic resonance imaging (fMRI). *IEEE Trans. Biomed. Eng, 51*, 966-970.

[15] Bagarinao, E., Matsuo, K. and Nakai, T. (2003) Real-time functional MRI using a PC cluster. *Concepts in Magnetic Resonance Part B-Magnetic Resonance Engineering, 19B*, 14-25.

[16] Mathiak, K. and Posse, S. (2001) Evaluation of motion and realignment for functional magnetic resonance imaging in real time. *Magn. Reson. Med., 45*, 167-171.

[17] deCharms, R. C., Christoff, K., Glover, G. H., Pauly, J. M., Whitfield, S. and Gabrieli, J. D. E. (2004) Learned regulation of spatially localized brain activation using real-time fMRI. *NeuroImage, 21*, 436-443.

[18] Frank, J. A., Ostuni, J. L., Yang, Y., Shiferaw, Y., Patel, A., Qin, J., Mattay, V. S., Lewis, B. K., Levin, R. L. and Duyn, J. H. (1999) Technical solution for an interactive functional MR imaging

examination: application to a physiologic interview and the study of cerebral physiology. *Radiology, 210*, 260-268.

[19] Jackson, J. I., Meyer, C. H., Nishimura, D. G. and Macovski, A. (1991) Selection of A Convolution Function for Fourier Inversion Using Gridding. *IEEE Transactions on Medical Imaging, 10*, 473-478.

[20] Goddard, N. H., Hood, G., Cohen, J. D., Eddy, W. F., Genovese, C. R., Noll, D. C. and Nystrom, L. E. (1997) Online analysis of functional MRI datasets on parallel platforms. *Journal of Supercomputing, 11*, 295-318.

[21] Friston, K. J., Williams, S., Howard, R., Frackowiak, R. S. and Turner, R. (1996) Movement-related effects in fMRI time-series. *Magn. Reson. Med., 35*, 346-355.

[22] Hajnal, J. V., Myers, R., Oatridge, A., Schwieso, J. E., Young, I. R. and Bydder, G. M. (1994) Artifacts due to stimulus correlated motion in functional imaging of the brain. *Magn. Reson. Med., 31*, 283-291.

[23] Cox, R. W. and Jesmanowicz, A. (1999) Real-time 3D image registration for functional MRI. *Magn Reson.Med., 42*, 1014-1018.

[24] Cox, R. W. (1996) *Motion and funcitonal MRI: Informal notes for the Boston '96 workshop on functional MRI* Available from http://afni.nimh.nih.gov/old/afni/regnotes.ps

[25] Frackowiak, R. S., Friston, K. J., Firth, C. D., Dolan, R. J., Price, C. J., Zeki, S., Ashburner, J. and Penny, W. (2004) *Human brain function* (second edition). San Diego:Academic Press.

[26] Thesen, S., Heid, O., Mueller, E. and Schad, L. R. (2000) Prospective acquisition correction for head motion with image-based tracking for real-time fMRI. *Magn. Reson. Med., 44*, 457-465.

[27] Hajnal, J. V., Saeed, N., Soar, E. J., Oatridge, A., Young, I. R. and Bydder, G. M. (1995) A registration and interpolation procedure for subvoxel matching of serially acquired MR images. *J. Comput. Assist. Tomogr., 19*, 289-296.

[28] Press, W. H., Teukolsky, S. A., Vetterling, W. T. and Flannery, B. P. (2002) *Numerical recipes in C++: The art of scientific computing* (second edition). Cambridge:Cambridge University Press.

[29] Friston, K. J., Ashburner, J., Frith, C. D., Poline, J. B., Heather, J. D. and Frackowiak, R. S. J. (1995) Spatial registration and normalization of images. *Human Brain Mapping, 3*, 165-189.

[30] Eddy, W. F., Fitzgerald, M. and Noll, D. C. (1996) Improved image registration by using Fourier interpolation. *Magn. Reson. Med., 36*, 923-931.

[31] Thesen, S., Henselmans, N. and Schad, L. R. (2000) BOLD Magnetic resonance imaging in real time. *Electromedica, 68*, 45-52.

[32] Tong, R. and Cox, R. W. (1999) Rotation of NMR images using the 2D chirp-z transform. *Magn. Reson. Med., 41*, 253-256.

[33] McKeown, M. J., Makeig, S., Brown, G. G., Jung, T. P., Kindermann, S. S., Bell, A. J. and Sejnowski, T. J. (1998) Analysis of fMRI data by blind separation into independent spatial components. *Human Brain Mapping, 6*, 160-88.

[34] McIntosh, A. R., Bookstein, F. L., Haxby, J. V. and Grady, C. L. (1996) Spatial pattern analysis of functional brain images using partial least squares. *NeuroImage, 3*, 143-57.

[35] Gembris, D., Taylor, J. G., Schor, S., Frings, W., Suter, D. and Posse, S. (2000) Functional magnetic resonance imaging in real time (FIRE): sliding-window correlation analysis and reference-vector optimization. *Magn. Reson.Med., 43*, 259-268.

[36] Posse, S., Fitzgerald, D., Gao, K., Habel, U., Rosenberg, D., Moore, G. J. and Schneider, F. (2003) Real-time fMRI of temporolimbic regions detects amygdala activation during single-trial self-induced sadness. *NeuroImage, 18*, 760-768.

[37] Cox, R. W., Jesmanowicz, A. and Hyde, J. S. (1995) Real-time functional magnetic resonance imaging. *Magnetic Resonance in Medicine, 33*, 230-6.

[38] Voyvodic, J. T. (1999) Real-time fMRI paradigm control, physiology, and behavior combined with near real-time statistical analysis. *NeuroImage, 10*, 91-106.

[39] Smyser, C., Grabowski, T. J., Frank, R. J., Haller, J. W. and Bolinger, L. (2001) Real-time multiple linear regression for fMRI supported by time-aware acquisition and processing. *Magn. Reson.Med., 45*, 289-298.

[40] Bagarinao, E., Matsuo, K., Nakai, T. and Sato, S. (2003) Estimation of general linear model coefficients for real-time application. *NeuroImage, 19*, 422-429.

[41] Esposito, F., Seifritz, E., Formisano, E., Morrone, R., Scarabino, T., Tedeschi, G., Cirillo, S., Goebel, R. and Di Salle, F. (2003) Real-time independent component analysis of fMRI time-series. *NeuroImage, 20*, 2209-2224.

[42] Hall, L. and Johansson, P. (2003) Neurofeedback and metacognition *Proceedings of 11th Int. Conference on Artificial Intelligence in Education AIED 2003 Supplementary Proceedings: Metacognition and Self-regulation in Learning with Metacognitive Tools*, 541-556.

[43] Jiang, A. P., Kennedy, D. N., Baker, J. R., Weisskoff, R. M., Tootell, R. B. H., Woods, R. P., Benson, R. R., Kwong, K. K., Brady, T. J., Rosen, B. R. and Belliveau, J. W. (1995) Motion detection and correction in functional MR imaging. *Human Brain Mapping, 3*, 224-235.

[44] Maas, L. C., Frederick, B. D. and Renshaw, P. F. (1997) Decoupled automated rotational and translational registration for functional MRI time series data: the DART registration algorithm. *Magn. Reson. Med., 37*, 131-139.

[45] Woods, R. P., Cherry, S. R. and Mazziotta, J. C. (1992) Rapid automated algorithm for aligning and reslicing PET images. *J. Comput. Assist. Tomogr., 16*, 620-633.

[46] Lee, C. C., Jack, C. R., Jr., Grimm, R. C., Rossman, P. J., Felmlee, J. P., Ehman, R. L. and Riederer, S. J. (1996) Real-time adaptive motion correction in functional MRI. *Magn. Reson. Med., 36*, 436-444.

[47] Derbyshire, J. A., Wright, G. A., Henkelman, R. M. and Hinks, R. S. (1998) Dynamic scan-plane tracking using MR position monitoring. *J. Magn. Reson. Imaging, 8*, 924-932.

[48] Lee, C. C., Grimm, R. C., Manduca, A., Felmlee, J. P., Ehman, R. L., Riederer, S. J. and Jack, C. R., Jr. (1998) A prospective approach to correct for inter-image head rotation in fMRI. *Magn. Reson. Med., 39*, 234-243.

[49] Ward, H. A., Riederer, S. J., Grimm, R. C., Ehman, R. L., Felmlee, J. P. and Jack, C. R., Jr. (2000) Prospective multiaxial motion correction for fMRI. *Magnetic Resonance in Medicine, 43*, 459-69.

[50] Ward, H. A., Riederer, S. J. and Jack, C. R., Jr. (2002) Real-time autoshimming for echo planar timecourse imaging. *Magn. Reson. Med., 48*, 771-780.

[51] Muresan, L., Renken, R., Roerdink, J. B. and Duifhuis, H. (2002) Position-history and spin-history artifacts in fMRI time series, *Proceedings of SPIE 4683*, San Diego, CA, USA, 444-451.

[52] Yang, S., Ross, T. J., Zhang, Y., Feng, H., Stien, E. A. and Yang, Y. (2004) Head-motion suppression using real-time feedback of motion curves and its effects on performance of task in fMRI. *Proceedings of 12th scientific meeting of the International Society for Magnetic Resonance in Medicine (ISMRM),* Kyoto, Japan.

[53] Goebel, R., Sorger, B., Birbaumer, N. and Weiskopf, N. (2005) Learning to play BOLD Brain Pong: From individual neurofeedback training to brain-brain interactions. *Proceedings of 11th annual meeting of the Organization for Human Brain Mapping,* Toronto, Canada.

[54] Maeda, F., Lutomski, L., MacLeod, S., Soneji, D., Mackey, S., Gabrieli, J. D. E., Glover, G. H., Pauly, J. M. and deCharms, R. C. (2005) Learned control over brain activation and pain in chronic pain patients achieved through repetitive training using real time fMRI (rtfMRI). *Proceedings of 11th annual meeting of the Organization for Human Brain Mapping,* Toronto, Canada.

INDEX

B

C

D

E

F

G

H

I

J

K

L

M

N

O

P

Q

R

S

T

U

V

W

Y